INTENSIVE HEALING DIETS

**PREVENTION'S LIBRARY
OF MEDICAL CARE AND NATURAL HEALING**™

INTENSIVE HEALING DIETS

by the Editors of Prevention®
Magazine Health Books

Rodale Press, Emmaus, Pennsylvania

Printed in the United States of America on recycled paper containing a high percentage of de-inked fiber.

Library of Congress Cataloging-in-Publication Data

Intensive healing diets / by the editors of Prevention magazine health books.

p.   cm. — (Prevention's library of medical care and natural healing)
Includes index.
ISBN 0-87857-786-6
1. Nutrition.   2. Nutritionally induced diseases—Prevention.   3. Diet therapy.   I. Prevention (Emmaus, Pa.)   II. Series.
RA784.I58   1988
615.8'54—dc19   88-15718
                                                         CIP

2 4 6 8 10 9 7 5 3 1   hardcover

NOTICE

This book is intended as a reference volume only, not as a medical manual or a guide to self-treatment. If you suspect that you have a medical problem, we urge you to seek competent medical help. Keep in mind that nutritional and health needs vary from person to person, depending on age, sex, health status and total diet. The information here is intended to help you make informed decisions about your health, not as a substitute for any treatment that may have been prescribed by your doctor.

PREVENTION'S LIBRARY OF MEDICAL CARE AND NATURAL HEALING™

Intensive Healing Diets **Editors:** William Gottlieb, Carol Keough, John Feltman, Mark Bricklin

Writing Contributions

Kim Anderson
James Anderson, Denis Burkitt, Constipation, Heart Disease, Recuperation, Vegetarianism

Don Barone
Allergies, Diabetes, Headaches, Immunity, Nathan Pritikin, Stroke, Ulcers

Alice Feinstein
Cancer, Dental Problems, High Blood Pressure, Impotence, Indigestion, Sippy and the Bland Diet

Karen Feridun
The Master Healing Diet

Marcia Holman
Anemia, Cystitis, Fibrocystic Breast Disease, Osteoporosis

Judith Lin
Arthritis, Diverticulosis, Gout, Insomnia, Walter Kempner and the Rice Diet, Medical Care and Your Healing Diet

Jeff Meade
The Psychology of Intensive Healing

Lisa Messinger
Diet and World Health, Lactose Intolerance, Overweight

Ellen Michaud
Celiac Disease

Cathy Perlmutter
Natural Food Advocates

Russell Wild
Cholesterol, Energy, Fringe Diets and Beyond, Nutritional Balance and Your Healing Diet, Nutritionists, Triglycerides

CONTENTS

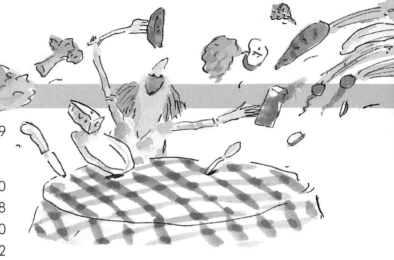

Eat light to be lively. See p. 67.

Staying happy, getting healthy. See p. 144.

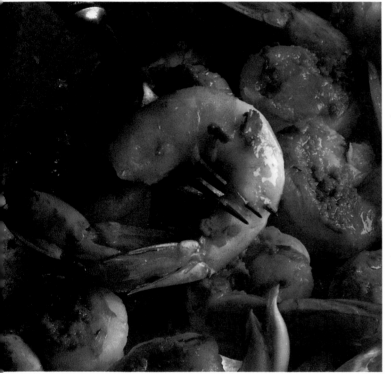

Enjoying the beneficial fish oils. See p. 47.

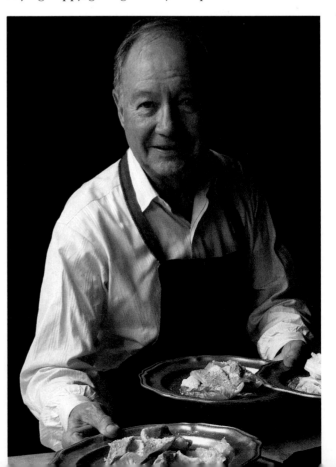

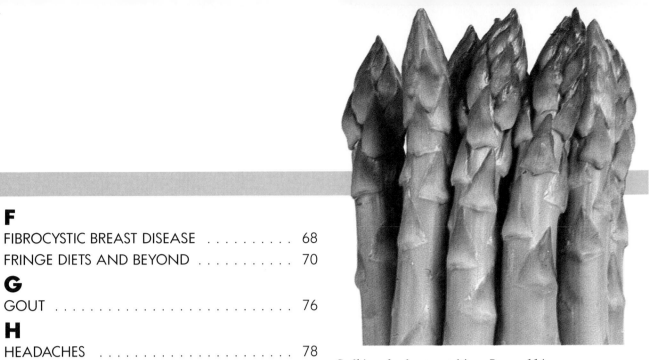

Stalking the best nutrition. See p. 114.

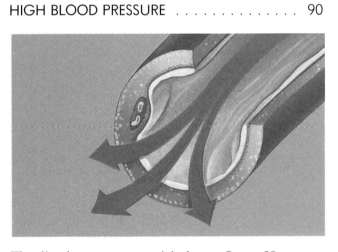

The diet that reverses arterial plaque. See p. 38.

PREFACE THE NEW SCIENCE OF CURATIVE NUTRITION

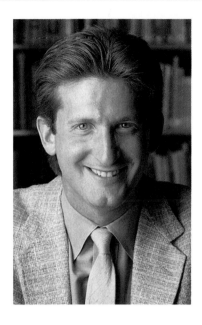

It's the place you never want to be—but where you'd be grateful to go if you'd just been in a serious car accident or had had a heart attack. It's the Intensive Care Unit, the concentrated core of the hospital, the part of the medical system where the best in healing technology—the beeping monitors, the hissing resuscitators, the drugs, the X-rays, the diagnoses—is focused on one thing: keeping you alive.

But the healing hardware in the Intensive Care Unit is second-rate compared to what you've got in your kitchen.

No, we're not talking about a new microwave that doubles as a heart monitor. We're talking about your *refrigerator*. Take that broccoli in the crisper, for example—it can help heal disease processes that may lead to arthritis, cancer, heart disease, high blood pressure and stroke. Ditto for the fish that's stored in the freezer. And if you've got some dried beans in the pantry, a bunch of bananas ripening on the counter, a loaf of whole wheat in the breadbox, some olive oil alongside the stove—well, then your kitchen is equipped with the best life-support system money can buy: the Intensive Healing Diet.

Yet, eating a healing diet doesn't mean being a food fanatic. Healing food, remember, is *intense*. Small amounts make big differences. For instance:

• When researchers from the State University of New York at Buffalo looked at the dietary history of people with lung cancer and people free of the disease, they found one important difference—the people without cancer had eaten about 7,000 more international units of vitamin A every day: the amount in *one* carrot.

• A 12-year study by medical researchers from California and England found that people whose daily diets contained an extra 400 milligrams of potassium had a 40 percent lower risk of death from stroke. That's the amount of potassium in *one* potato.

• In a study from West Germany, researchers found that eating fish lowered cholesterol and high blood pressure. Not eating fish every day. Not even every other day. Just three times a week.

This book is filled with hundreds more examples of the power of food to prevent or cure health problems. It provides you with the facts and inspiration you need to get the best kind of intensive care—the self-care of an intensive healing diet. Read it—and use it—in good health.

William Gottlieb
Editorial Director, Prevention® Magazine Health Books

ALLERGIES

Boy, that lobster looks good. Sitting there on the bed of lettuce, it's so fresh you swear you can still see the ocean in its eyes.

As the waiter adjusts your plastic bib, you crack one of the lobster's claws. Then you take the little fork and pull out one tiny white morsel of the ever-so-sweet meat.

Delicately, you dip it into the silver cup of butter, twirling it so that every thread is covered. Rarely do you have the nerve to order from the big-time side of the menu, but soon the payoff will come; soon your taste buds will explode.

Ahhhhhhh, there's no other taste quite like it. "Maybe the rat race is worth it after all," you think as you sit back and enjoy.

Then it hits. Suddenly your body is covered by hundreds of red hives, and your skin starts taking on the color of the lobster you just ate. You start to scratch, itching everywhere. Your nose becomes plugged, and you start to wheeze. Your throat swells up, and you feel a tightness in your chest.

All this, and you haven't even been given the dinner check yet, so you know it's not a reaction to the current price of lobster. The shock to your system is probably coming not from the cost of your meal but from what you're eating. If you love lobster but it hates you, you may have a food allergy.

"For the most part, a person who has a food allergy has a dramatic reaction—sometimes even life-threatening—to food immediately," says William

FOOD ALLERGIES CHANGE WITH AGE

Some things you *do* outgrow. Compare the foods that cause allergy problems in adults with those that affect children under three. You'll see that as you mature, so do your allergies.

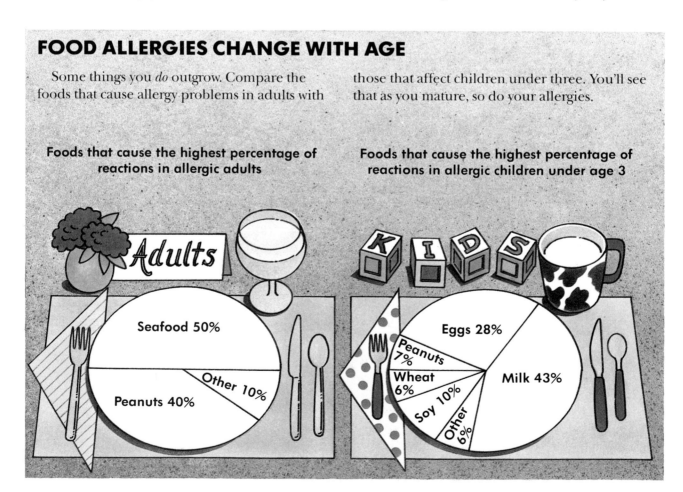

Foods that cause the highest percentage of reactions in allergic adults

Seafood 50%
Peanuts 40%
Other 10%

Foods that cause the highest percentage of reactions in allergic children under age 3

Eggs 28%
Peanuts 7%
Wheat 6%
Soy 10%
Other 6%
Milk 43%

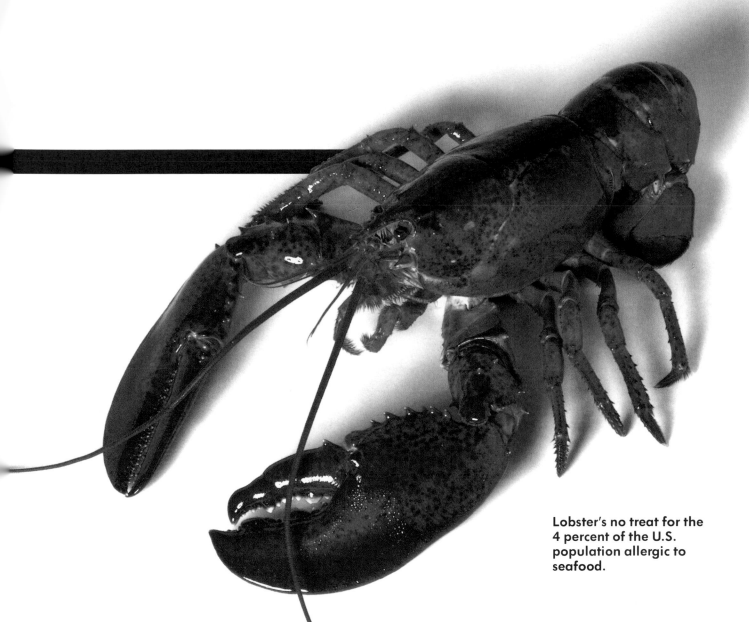

Lobster's no treat for the 4 percent of the U.S. population allergic to seafood.

Ziering, M.D., an allergist in California. "By 'immediately' we mean within an hour or so. It can be within seconds or minutes of eating the food, but normally if it doesn't occur within an hour, it's unlikely that your reaction is based on what you ate." Dr. Ziering adds that some people can suffer from "late-onset reactions"—where their reactions don't occur for 12 hours or more. Delayed allergic reactions occur less often and tend to be less severe.

Whether it's right after lunch or nearing midnight, that awful attack can be brought on by almost any food. One man's wheat, it seems, is another man's wheeze.

Robert Dockhorn, M.D., an allergist and chairman of the Food Allergy Committee of the American College of Allergists, says, however, that *some* foods do cause more problems than others. "Some of the basic foods—like milk, eggs, wheat and corn—are those that tend to cause the continual, ongoing reactions. The legume group of foods, like peanuts and soy, also cause lots of adverse reactions in people. And there are many people who have problems with chocolate, citrus or seafood."

Yes, there's danger lurking in the deep, too. Experts say that as many as 4 percent of the U.S. population may be allergic to seafood. Most people who are allergic to seafood should avoid eating lobster, shrimp, crabs and oysters. New research, however, is reeling in problems other than shellfish. "Fish are showing up as a problem in some people," says Robert Bush, M.D., associate professor of medicine at the University of Wisconsin and chief of allergy at the Veterans Hospital in Madison.

"Codfish allergies are starting to rank pretty high worldwide. In Scandinavia, codfish is the major food allergy in adults."

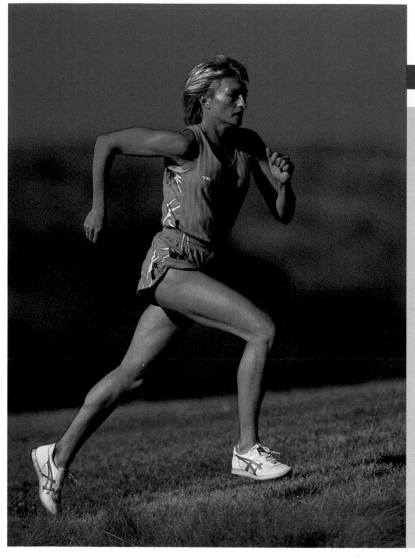

Dr. Ziering adds that people in this country are also affected. "Grouper fish or snapper will cause a reaction in some people. Within a few hours after eating, they will start to have itchy skin, a headache and an upset stomach."

THE CASE OF THE HONEYDEW HIVES

At times—literally—food allergies just come and go. One time you react to a food, and the next time you don't. The situation is rather mysterious.

Get out your trenchcoat, it's time to play a little detective. Say it's January, and by some outrageous stroke of luck, you found a honeydew melon in the produce section of your supermarket. After forking over all of your money, plus a few promissory notes, you brought it home and ate it for breakfast. No

problem. Or so you think.

Now, flip the calendar ahead a few months. It's September or October, there's a touch of Indian summer in the air and there's more than just a touch of ragweed wafting in that same breeze. You're back in the supermarket, and lo and behold, so are the honeydews. This time you can buy ten for the price of that one January melon.

You take your bag of honeydews home and, sitting out on your porch, you read the paper and eat a little of the 'dew.

Gesundheit. Bless you. You need a tissue? Why all the sneezes? For that matter, why all the hives? Yesterday you felt fine, so why the problem today?

You may be suffering from a *combination* of things. "Mixing ragweed with melons can cause an

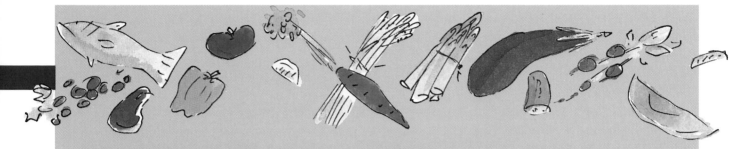

WELCOME TO THE ALLERGY FAMILY

If Mr. and Mrs. Cran Berry tend to get under your skin, chances are their little offshoots, Blue and Huckle, will give you the same reaction. Here are some foods and their relatives to watch out for.

FAMILY	PLANT FOODS
APPLE	Apple, crabapple, pear, quince
BUCKWHEAT	Buckwheat, garden sorrel, rhubarb
CASHEW	Cashew, mango, pistachio
CHOCOLATE	Chocolate (cocoa), cola, gum karaya
CITRUS	Citron, grapefruit, kumquat, lemon, lime, orange, tangerine
COMPOSITE	Artichoke, camomile, chicory, dandelion, lettuce, escarole
GINGER	Cardamom, ginger, turmeric
GRAIN	Barley, corn, millet, oats, rice, rye, sugar cane, wheat
LAUREL	Avocado, bay leaf, cinnamon, sassafras
LEGUME	Alfalfa, bean, carob, guar gum, licorice, pea, peanut
LILY	Asparagus, chive, garlic, leek, onion, sarsaparilla
MELON	Cantaloupe, cucumber, gherkin, honeydew, pumpkin, squash
MINT	Basil, catnip, oregano, peppermint, sage, spearmint, thyme
MULBERRY	Breadfruit, fig, mulberry
MUSTARD	Broccoli, brussels sprouts, cabbage, horseradish, radish, turnip
PARSLEY	Carrot, celery, parsnip
POTATO	Eggplant, green and red pepper, paprika, tobacco, tomato
WALNUT	Black walnut, butternut, English walnut, hickory nut, pecan

FAMILY	ANIMAL FOODS
BOVINE	Beef cattle (including veal), buffalo, lamb, and their milk
FLOUNDER	Dab, halibut, plaice, sole, turbot
LOBSTER	Crayfish, langostino, lobster
PHEASANT	Chicken, Cornish hen, peafowl, quail, and their eggs
SALMON	All salmon species, all trout species
SHRIMP	Prawn, shrimp

FOODS WITHOUT RELATIVES

Catfish	Kiwi	Pineapple	Squirrel
Coffee	Maple sugar	Poppyseed	Swordfish
Crab	Nutmeg	Rabbit	Tapioca
Grape	Olive	Saffron	Tea
Hog	Oyster	Scallop	Vanilla
Honey	Papaya	Sesame seed	Whitefish

adverse reaction in some people," says Dr. Dockhorn. "Some people can't eat honeydews or cantaloupe during the fall when they are exposed to ragweed. During other times of the year, they can eat melons and not have a problem. It's the addition of ragweed that causes them to have an adverse reaction."

CRAVING A SNEEZE

You know that chocolate makes you wheeze, but sometimes you get such a craving for it that you've got to have *just a little bite*. Despite all common sense, you dig in. Why?

Yes, that tiny shrimp causes you big trouble, but you have such a craving for scampi, you have to eat it just this one time. Hives or not.

Many times, people actually crave what's worst for them, allergists say, and this is a good clue to finding out what you're allergic to. "Some people say that they just have to have eight glasses a milk a day," says Dr. Ziering, "or they eat lots of candy bars or cookies. Whenever we hear someone saying they're addicted to certain foods, it truly is an addiction. Allergists have learned to suspect an allergy when a person craves certain foods and is continually hungering for them. During this 'avoidance period' the victim actually experiences withdrawal symptoms, which build up until they eat the offending food again," the doctor explains.

If what you eat gives you a rash, chances are you should also get a RAST. Dr. Dockhorn says the new RAST test, which is a laboratory blood test, seems to be a better way of searching for food allergies than the old skin test. "There are a lot of problems with skin testing for food sensitivities, basically because many of the extracts we use for skin testing are not that accurate. You also get lots of interference from irritation and from injecting the food extract under the skin. By doing the RAST test, you can look for IgE antibodies to foods," explains Dr. Dockhorn. (IgE antibodies are the substances that produce allergic reactions.) "I think it's a better evaluation for food sensitivities than skin testing," he says. The test can show if you're allergic to pea-

nuts or fish or more than 25 other foods.

If food addictions and a RAST test don't uncover the culprit, there's a third alternative—the elimination diet.

A PROCESS OF ELIMINATION

Think of the world as a supermarket. If every time you walked down the dairy aisle, you broke out in hives and started sneezing, chances are that you and your shopping cart wouldn't go past that section anymore.

Such immediate responses are easy to see—once your eyes stop tearing. But what if nothing happened until you were in the checkout line, *after* you had been through the whole store. Which aisle, which food, was the culprit?

"An elimination diet is one of many ways to uncover a food sensitivity," says Dr. Dockhorn. How does it work?

Say, for instance, that once a week for the last few years you've made sloppy joes out of ground unicorn. (They taste pretty good, except for having a slightly mystical flavor.) It's no mystery, though, that shortly after eating them, you start to sneeze, break out in hives and look for a gnome to kick. But what's causing this reaction, the unicorn meat or the powdered hummingbird tongue that you spice it with? Here's where the elimination diet starts. "Remove the food that you suspect from your diet for two or three weeks," says Dr. Ziering. "See if, in fact, you do feel a lot better. If you haven't had the symptoms for that time period, now's the time to check.

"Take the suspect food and challenge your system with it. [Be sure you let your doctor know what you're up to.] Put it back into your diet in extra amounts for a four- or five-day period. If this 'challenge' test provokes the symptoms—if the hives or sneezing comes back—then that food looks highly suspicious.

"To be sure that you're having an adverse reaction to *that* food, eliminate the food from your diet one more time; then at a later date, try it again. If the same reaction occurs, you can be reasonably sure that you've found the problem," says Dr. Ziering.

ALLERGIES
A DAY OF INTENSIVE HEALING

A.M.

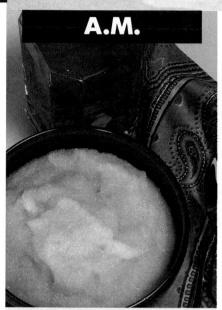

Cranberry juice
Cream of Rice cereal,
cooked with apple juice
and cinnamon
Hot cider

NOON

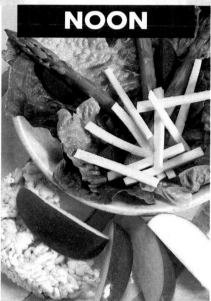

Vegetarian onion soup with
buckwheat groats or
kernels
Vegetable salad (romaine,
pickled beets, raw sweet
potato sticks and
asparagus)
Rice cakes
Sparkling water
Apple wedges

P.M.

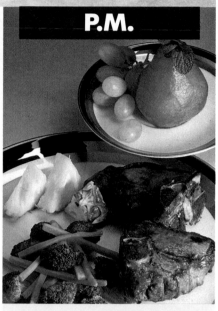

Fresh pineapple wedges
Broiled lamb chops
Boiled or baked potato
Stir-fried julienne carrots
and broccoli
Poached pear in cranapple
juice with green grape
garnish
Sparkling water

DISASTER PLATE

Shrimp salad with
mayonnaise
Whole wheat bread
Tomato wedges
Corn on the cob
Hot cocoa

If you see this particular
meal listed as the daily

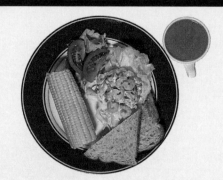

special, beware. It could
cause those with food allergies special problems. You
may want to avoid seafood,
a common allergen. And if
you have an allergy to
milk, look for it hidden in
foods like bread or hot
cocoa.

INTENSIVE HEALING RECIPE:
ALLERGIES

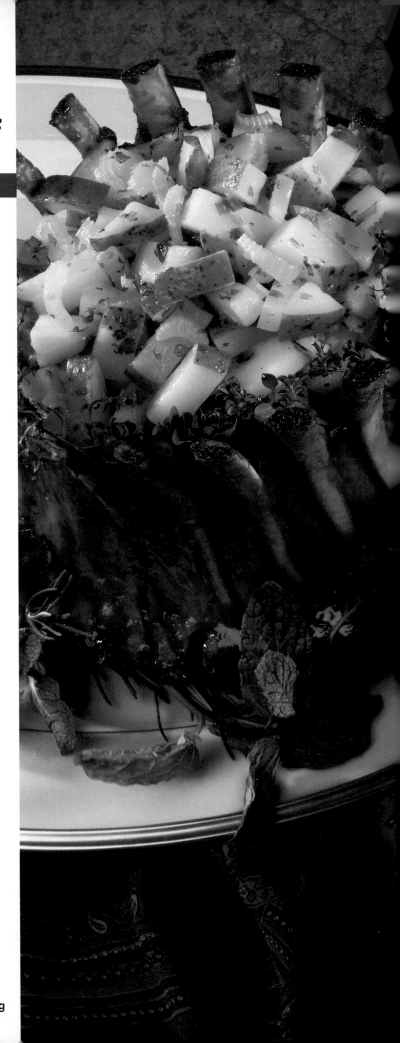

Lamb is an excellent choice, because even among those who have allergies, this food rarely causes trouble.

CROWN ROAST OF LAMB WITH POTATO STUFFING

Roast

1   crown roast of lamb (3½ to 4 lb.)
2   cloves garlic, cut into slivers
2   tsp. olive oil
2   tsp. lemon juice
1   tsp. minced fresh rosemary or ½ tsp. crumbled dried rosemary

Stuffing

4   cups diced potatoes
1   Tbsp. olive oil
⅓   cup minced scallions
½   cup thinly sliced celery
1   bay leaf
1   tsp. minced fresh thyme or ½ tsp. dried thyme
¼   cup minced parsley
1   Tbsp. minced chives

Preheat the oven to 425°F.

To make the roast: Wipe roast with paper towels and place on a rack in a roasting pan. With a small knife, cut slits in roast and insert garlic.

In a small bowl, combine oil, lemon juice and rosemary, then rub mixture all over roast. Cover bone tips with small pieces of aluminum foil and insert a meat thermometer into roast, making sure it doesn't touch bone.

Place roast in the oven and bake for 15 minutes. Reduce heat to 325°F and continue baking for about 1 hour. For medium-rare meat (150°F on meat thermometer), bake 15 to 17 minutes per pound; for medium meat (160°F), bake 18 to 20 minutes per pound.

To make the stuffing: In a large saucepan, steam or boil potatoes until tender, about 5 minutes. Set aside.

Heat oil in a medium-size skillet. Add scallions, celery, bay leaf, thyme and parsley and cook about 6 minutes, or until vegetables are soft, stirring occasionally. Remove bay leaf. Add potatoes and chives and heat through. Remove from heat and keep warm.

When roast is done, place on a serving platter and let stand for 10 minutes before carving. Remove aluminum foil and spoon some stuffing into center of roast.

Yield: 4 to 6 servings

Crown Roast of Lamb with Potato Stuffing

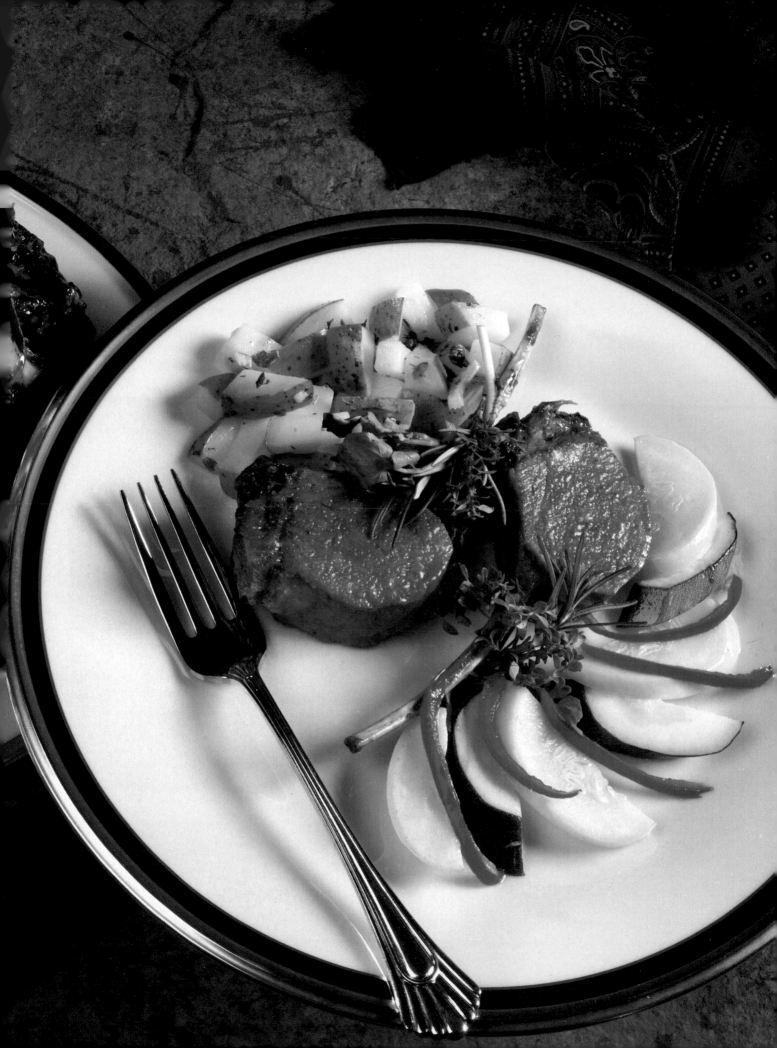

JAMES ANDERSON

ew York City, 9:00 A.M.—A distinguished senior executive, despite his years still fit and trim through regular hard exercise, sits on the terrace adjoining his Fifth Avenue apartment. Gazing out over Central Park's lush greenery, he pours milk into a bowl of sliced fresh fruit.

Chicago, 7:00 A.M.—An attractive young woman, fresh from her morning run, moves briskly through her kitchen collecting the wherewithal for a nourishing breakfast: skim milk, brown sugar and oatmeal. Sweating lightly, she frees one hand to adjust her headband and then walks toward the stove.

San Francisco, 5:00 A.M.—A battered old sea captain sits below-deck at a table that resembles him—nicked and chipped but still rock-steady. The solid old fishing boat creaks and groans with each roll of the sea, and in the dim yellow light of an ancient brass lantern, the captain sprinkles bran over his cereal—a heavy dusting of fine brown fiber.

What do the three have in common? Very little

—except a commitment to protecting their health through better nutrition. All three make it a point to get more fiber from their food—and for that, one man can take most of the credit: the University of Kentucky's James Anderson, M.D., a physician who is generally recognized as the "father of fiber" in the United States.

THE OAT-BRAN MAN: PROFILE OF A WINNER

James Anderson, M.D., was born August 6, 1936, in Hinton, West Virginia. Early on, he picked the career that would eventually lead him to international recognition.

"My mother was a nurse in a small town, and I just always wanted to be a doctor. Even when other kids wanted to be firemen and pilots, I still wanted to be a doctor," Dr. Anderson says.

In a hurry to do it, he whipped through undergraduate training, medical school and internship/

A HIGH-FIBER DIET LOWERS INSULIN NEEDS

Large amounts of what used to be called roughage in your diet won't just make you regular—it will improve your body's ability to burn sugar. In one study, 12 lean men with

adult-onset diabetes were able to reduce and in some cases stop insulin injections after being on Dr. Anderson's diet.

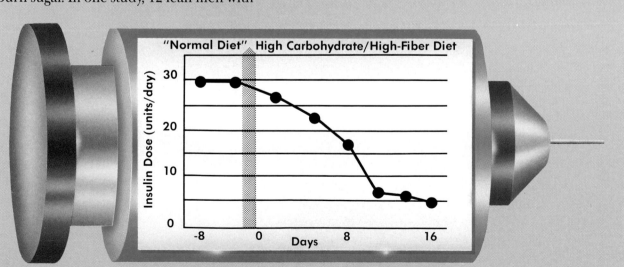

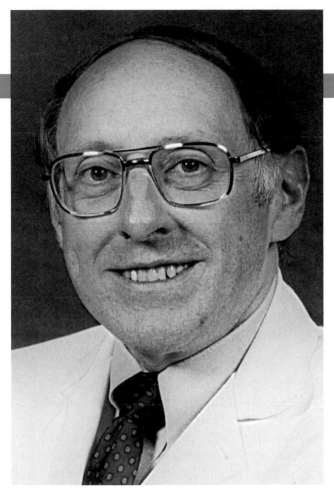

Dr. James Anderson, professor of medicine and clinical nutrition at the University of Kentucky's College of Medicine, held a leadership position in early research, exploring the role of fiber in human health. He played a key part in publicizing the result: Fiber's good for you.

residency at the prestigious Mayo Clinic before going to work for the U.S. Army as chief of Fitzsimmons Hospital's Metabolic-Renal Section. Early on, he became interested in the disease he'd build his career around—diabetes.

"In medical school, I saw an opportunity there [in diabetes] for self-help. The traditional approach —the physician prescribed, the patient complied— didn't work well with the disease because it fluctuates so much from day to day. The physician can coach, but diabetics need to be able to change plays at the line of scrimmage. Most of them lacked the skills to do that. I perceived that as an area where, especially with diet, I could make a contribution."

And contribute he did. Dr. Anderson today is internationally recognized for the result of that initial interest—a diet that helps diabetics control their disease with the absolute minimum of outside medical help. And he is widely credited with making the American public aware of fiber's importance to health.

The meal plan that did all that is called the HCF (high-carbohydrate, high-fiber) diet. People using it get 55 to 60 percent of their energy from carbohydrates, 15 to 20 percent from protein and the final 20 to 25 percent from fat. In the process, they also eat 50 or more grams of fiber.

The diet works, and works well—a fact that Dr. Anderson and his associates have thoroughly documented. HCF diets consistently reduce insulin requirements, improve glycemic (blood sugar) control and drive cholesterol and triglyceride (blood fats) levels down—effects that benefit both diabetics and nondiabetics.

Dr. Anderson says the high-carbohydrate component evolved out of work on field rations for the army: It improved a soldier's ability to burn sugar, which led to further research on diabetics.

But interestingly, the inclusion of fiber in the evolving diet came about largely by chance. "Like a lot of investigators, we got there partly by accident, by serendipity," Dr. Anderson laughingly says today.

"We had a nagging concern about triglycerides: The HC diets drove them up by 50 percent or so, when we really wanted to drive them down. That's where fiber came in: We read a medical report that said wheat bran lowered triglycerides. We tried it, and it worked."

Publication of papers based on his research and similar reports from other teams in the 1970s led to the present awareness of fiber's role in human health—a large one that has been thoroughly documented since then. Dr. Anderson continues his work with diabetics today, but he is exploring a new avenue: the role of soluble fiber—psyllium (Metamucil) and oats in particular—in lowering cholesterol levels. The indications at this time are that it works.

ANEMIA

Fatigue. Being tired *all the time*—that's fatigue. "I used to just lie down on the floor wherever I was and go to sleep," is the way one woman described her extreme tiredness. "I remember my neighbors walking in and thinking I was dead."

Why is this woman a zombie? Anemia put a hex on her blood.

In anemia, the red blood cells that transport oxygen are deficient in size and number. The cause can be a lack of folate, a B vitamin that helps control the genetic messages that form red blood cells. But the most common nutritional cause of anemia—particularly for women—is a diet low in iron. "It is estimated that in the United States, at least 20 percent of women of childbearing age are iron-deficient," says Holly Atkinson, M.D., author of *Women and Fatigue.*

Iron is part of hemoglobin, the red blood cell component that actually hauls oxygen to the cells and tissues. Women of childbearing age need 18 milligrams of iron a day (men get by on 10). The problem, explains Marvin Adner, M.D., director of the Division of Hematology at Framingham Union Hospital in Massachusetts, is that many women are unable to meet this daily iron requirement for one reason or another. "They may have heavy menstrual periods that drain away iron, or they may be eating low-cal meals and skimping on iron-rich foods."

BEST FOOD SOURCES OF IRON

FOOD	PORTION	IRON (MG)
Chicken liver, cooked	3 oz.	7.20
Beef liver, fried	3 oz.	5.30
Soybeans, boiled	½ cup	4.40
Blackstrap molasses	1 Tbsp.	3.20
Spinach, cooked	½ cup	3.20
Rump roast, lean, cooked	3 oz.	3.10
Potato, baked	1	2.80
Tuna, canned in water	3 oz.	2.72
Sirloin steak, lean/fat	3 oz.	2.50
Sunflower seeds, dried	¼ cup	2.40
Lima beans, large, boiled	½ cup	2.30
Pistachio nuts, dried	¼ cup	2.20
Broccoli, cooked	1 spear	2.10
Cashew nuts, dry-roasted	¼ cup	2.10
Ground beef, extra lean, broiled, medium	3 oz.	2.00
Swiss chard, cooked	½ cup	2.00
Turkey, dark meat (without skin), cooked	3 oz.	2.00
Soybeans, dry-roasted	¼ cup	1.70
Beet greens, cooked	½ cup	1.40
Broccoli, raw	1 spear	1.30
Sesame seeds, whole, dried	1 Tbsp.	1.30
Prunes, dried, cooked	½ cup	1.20
Apricots, dried, sulfured, cooked	¼ cup	1.00
Raisins, seedless, packed	¼ cup	0.90
Spinach, raw, chopped	½ cup	0.80

EATING FOR IRON INSURANCE

The best way to bolster your blood cells is to beef up your meals with iron-rich foods and follow a few nutritional guidelines. Do that, says Dr. Adner, and you may "increase your hemoglobin and turn your anemia around quickly." Here's how to get the most iron out of your meals.

• Eat enough meat. Beef, pork, the dark meat of fowl and fish all contain heme iron, the kind your body readily absorbs. Vegetarians should have frequent servings of non-heme-iron foods like broccoli, dark green, leafy vegetables, blackstrap molasses, kidney beans, dried apricots and iron-fortified grains and cereals. (See the accompanying table for more iron sources.)

• Dish up vitamin C with each meal. According to food science expert Fergus Clydesdale, Ph.D., of the University of Massachusetts, a glass of orange juice or vitamin C-rich fruits or vegetables such as potatoes, cabbage, cantaloupe and broccoli, eaten with a meal (even a meatless one), may dramatically increase the iron absorption from foods.

• Guard against the iron robbers. Save your tea for teatime. Studies have found that tannic acid in tea can block iron absorption from meals by nearly two-thirds. And take your calcium supplements separately from iron sources—they also may inhibit iron absorption.

ANEMIA
A DAY OF INTENSIVE HEALING

A.M.

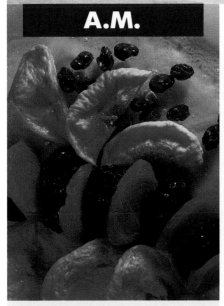

Prune juice
Sunflower-seed muffins
   made with blackstrap
   molasses
Dried fruit compote (prunes,
   raisins, apricots and
   peaches)
Turkey sausage patties
Hot beef tea

NOON

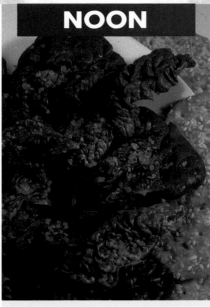

Beef, lentil and navy bean
   soup
Chicken liver pâté
Sesame wheat crackers
Spinach salad topped with
   wheat germ
Tomato juice cocktail

P.M.

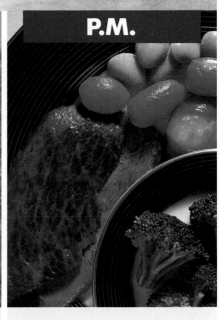

Pot roast, potatoes, carrots
   and lima beans (cooked
   in iron pot)
Marinated blanched broc-
   coli salad
Raisin bread
Fancy figs

DISASTER PLATE

Cottage cheese
Fruit salad (grapes, orange
   and grapefruit sections,
   kiwifruit and papaya)
Saltines
Milk

   If you gathered in one
meal the *worst* possible

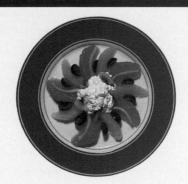

foods for someone with
anemia, the menu might
look like this list. Cottage
cheese and milk contain
very little iron. Saltines are
virtually without nutrition.
And while fresh fruit is
good, it offers little iron.

ARTHRITIS

Aah! Eee! Aiee! Ohh! Ooooo! Another entertaining evening spent reciting your vowel sounds? Oh, so sorry, but you've got arthritis, and such is tonight's oral accompaniment to the not-so-simple act of sitting down.

Darn right, you chide, hand on aching hip. What's more, there's not a thing you can do about it but keep a stiff upper lip—the last thing a body in your shape needs.

AN OCEAN OF RELIEF

Fish oil can ease the discomfort of arthritis, a study at Albany Medical College showed. For 14 weeks, 33 people with rheumatoid arthritis were given either fish-oil capsules or capsules containing an inactive substance (placebo). Nobody knew which they received. After a brief break, the capsules were switched for a second 14-week period. When given fish oil, patients showed an observable improvement in most symptoms. (In the table, a negative number indicates reduced occurrences of a symptom.)

	FISH OIL		PLACEBO	
	7 WKS.	14 WKS.	7 WKS.	14 WKS.
Morning stiffness (min.)	−2.7	−5.9	22.4	49.4
Time to fatigue (min.)	94.0	176.8	11.8	8.4
Grip strength measurement	−3.4	9.7	−2.0	2.9
Physician assessment of pain (0-4)	−0.06	−0.06	0.14	0.06
Patient assessment of pain (0-4)	−0.14	−0.21	−0.06	0.0
Physician overall assessment (0-4)	−0.17	−0.27	0.0	−0.9
Patient overall assessment (0-4)	−0.06	−0.11	−0.9	0.0
50-foot walking time (sec.)	−0.01	−0.22	0.39	0.39
Tender joints (num.)	−2.0	−3.5	−0.8	0.01
Swollen joints (num.)	−0.4	−2.8	−0.3	−1.0

Arthritis. It's a real pain—in the body's joints, specifically. Of the numerous forms it takes, osteoarthritis is the most common. This form is characterized by stiff joints that hurt like heck. Most of us will develop it sooner or later, but generally later, since it seems to be an inevitable companion to old age. Second most common is rheumatoid arthritis, which is highly painful and highly inflammatory. This form tends to strike younger people—the majority of them women—and to run an unpredictable course of comings and goings.

What causes arthritis? No one knows for sure. How you get rid of it is another riddle. But before you despair and repair to your sickbed for the duration, check out these hopeful hints offered by arthritis experts.

LOSE WEIGHT, STAND STRAIGHT

Art Mollen, D.O., a preventive medicine specialist, makes no bones about his treatment approach.

"I believe that weight loss is the cornerstone of treatment for arthritis. Excess weight puts excess stress and strain on all your joints, especially on your lower back, the part of the spine most susceptible to arthritis."

Studies show that taking off 20 pounds can cut your hurt in half, he says—even if you're carrying lots more excess fat than that. (This is good news, too, for those who don't yet show signs of osteoarthritis, because slimming down might even help prevent the disease from progressing.) The mere act of cutting calories from your diet can decrease arthritis inflammation. Studies in Japan have shown that sufferers placed on fasts could be relieved of many symptoms. Dr. Mollen places his own patients on a vegetable juice fast at least one day a week.

Try a low-fat diet to slowly but steadily dip down to your ideal weight. For help see the entry on overweight, beginning on page 138.

SOMETHING FISHY

Casting about for innovative ways to control the inflammation of rheumatoid arthritis, researchers

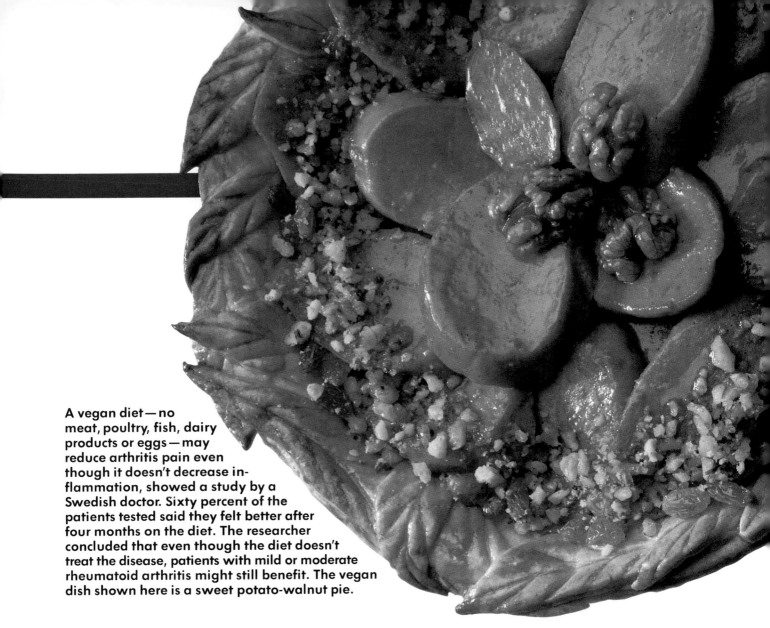

A vegan diet—no meat, poultry, fish, dairy products or eggs—may reduce arthritis pain even though it doesn't decrease inflammation, showed a study by a Swedish doctor. Sixty percent of the patients tested said they felt better after four months on the diet. The researcher concluded that even though the diet doesn't treat the disease, patients with mild or moderate rheumatoid arthritis might still benefit. The vegan dish shown here is a sweet potato-walnut pie.

are now catching on to the powers of omega-3, a futuristic-sounding substance that has actually been around for a long time. It's a class of fatty acid contained in fish oil.

"We have three tantalizing studies that have indicated a medical benefit from fish oil," says Richard Sperling, M.D., a rheumatologist from the Harvard School of Medicine who has conducted some of the primary research in the area.

Dr. Sperling and his colleagues are exploring activities in the body's immune system, our built-in defense department against disease. In rheumatoid arthritis, scientists think, the body somehow mistakes its own joints as foreign invaders that need to be driven out. Three internal pathways act something like ammunition factories, producing inflammatory chemicals and shooting them into the body's joints, which are left aching and swollen.

Leukotriene B_4 is one such chemical. In Dr. Sperling's study, rheumatoid arthritis patients were given fish-oil capsules over a period of six weeks. Lo and behold, their cells' ability to produce leukotriene decreased, along with some of their pain and inflammation. In a separate study, researchers found that fish oil also seemed to cut back on another inflammatory chemical called the platelet activating factor.

"There's no other drug with the effect of fish oil," says Dr. Sperling. "None of the other available drugs are known to block these important pathways."

While scientists continue to measure the effects of these interesting chemicals, rheumatoid arthritis sufferers certainly can't do themselves any harm by simply adding more fish to their diets.

FOOD FIGHT!

And then, some researchers say, there's the itchy matter of food allergies. Your favorite foods could

23

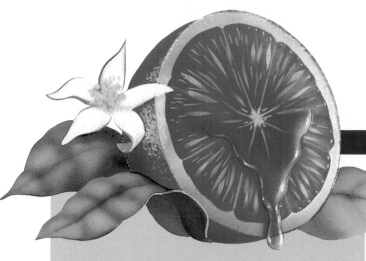

VITAMIN C—RUBBING IT IN

For the arthritis sufferer, getting an extra-healthy dose of vitamin C—essential for fending off infections and healing wounds—could be extra-important. For starters, people with arthritis tend to take a lot of aspirin, which depletes the body's vitamin C supply. Furthermore, research has shown that a large percentage of those with arthritis have an overall lower level of vitamin C in their blood, maybe because they use it up faster than other people.

At least one researcher is looking at a new way to enlist vitamin C in the battle against arthritis: Robert H. Davis, Ph.D., professor of physiology at Pennsylvania College of Podiatric Medicine, has high hopes for reducing rheumatoid arthritis inflammation by means of an ointment you apply to the skin over aching joints.

"My research in this area goes back to the late 1940s, when steroids were first being used to treat arthritis. They are effective, but they have serious side effects. I started to look around for a natural substance," he says.

Dr. Davis combined vitamin C with aloe vera and ribonucleic acid in an ointment and applied it to the arthritic paws of laboratory animals. Their swelling went down significantly.

This approach might actually help prevent the disease as well as treat it, Dr. Davis says. Currently, he is experimenting with other vitamin C combinations that the body might be able to absorb more efficiently.

"We've needed a breakthrough in rheumatoid arthritis for a long time," Dr. Davis says. "This is probably the best hope we have."

be a culprit in your arthritis, says Lyndon Mansfield, M.D., professor of medicine and head of the Division of Immunology and Allergy at Texas Tech University.

The problem, once again, involves the immune system, Dr. Mansfield explains. Certain foods are given the same unwarm welcome as other substances you might be allergic to—household dust, for example, or the neighborhood pollen patch.

Dr. Mansfield cites a study by Richard Panush, M.D., of the University of Florida College of Medicine. His subject was a person with arthritis who said her symptoms seemed to increase when she consumed milk, meat and beans. Over several weeks, researchers gave her capsules that, unknown to her, contained milk. Sure enough, her symptoms worsened. When she took milk-free capsules, her symptoms were absent.

Which foods might you be allergic to? "The foods likely to be problems are those that you eat a lot," says Dr. Mansfield. "In other words, your favorites." In a rather perverse manner, your body has a craving for the very foods it is allergic to, say some physicians—although this theory remains to be scientifically proven.

Take a look at your eating habits. If you see the same foods disappearing from your cupboards and into your mouth again and again, you could be allergic to them. You can be tested by a specialist to find out for sure. Or you might just remove the suspect food from your diet and see if, over a period of time, it makes a comforting difference in your arthritis symptoms. (For related information, see the discussion of the no-nightshades diet on page 70.)

YOUR DAILY DOSE

A number of specific vitamins and minerals—from vitamin C (see the accompanying box) to zinc—have been proposed for treating arthritis. The important thing is to get your daily requirement of all nutrients. If you feel you can't because grocery shopping and cooking are difficult, try to get help. Your health is in the balance.

KITCHEN HELPERS

Thanks to creative designers who have your special needs in mind, a variety of household tools are available to help you get a better grip on the practical challenges of nourishment, from slicing bread just right to doing a nifty clean-up act with one hand after dinner.

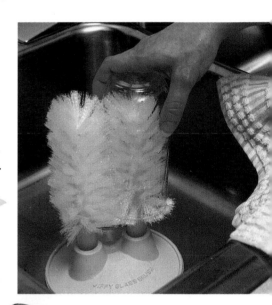

Meals become the pleasant experience they should be with the aid of utensils with oversized handles. Easier to grasp than ordinary silverware, these pieces maximize your hand or arm strength while minimizing discomfort.

No matter how you slice it, your bread comes out in neat pieces with this adjustable cutting board and easy-to-hold serrated knife.

This handy bottle brush attaches to your kitchen sink with suction cups. It allows you to hold glassware with both hands — reducing the risk of breakage.

Burned up over one too many overcooked meals? Relax with this large-size timer. Mounted on a wall or placed on your kitchen counter, it is easily set with a turn of your hand.

Don't drip a drop with these special grip mugs. The molded plastic handle is comfortable to grasp even when you have arthritis or a weak grip.

25

DENIS BURKITT

Imagine old Africa, in the time of the pharaohs, and a circle of warriors gathered around a fire. Fireflies embroider the night sky, red stars on a sheet of black velvet. In the distance, green hills shimmer silver in the moonlight. A faint rumble of drums rolls out over the plain; the warriors look up—and in the darkness, a lion roars.

Cut to the same meadow today.

Fireflies still embroider the night sky, red stars on a sheet of black velvet. In the distance, green hills shimmer silver in the moonlight. And in the darkness, a lion roars. But the bony and bespectacled English scientist sitting next to *this* fire ignores all to go on counting the day's catch: a fine collection of clear plastic bags holding splendidly large samples of what the Chinese politely call night soil. The rest of the world calls it . . . well, *stool*.

The work of Denis Burkitt, M.D., in modern Africa may lack the romance of ancient Africa, but it replaces it with something more important: medical significance.

Dr. Burkitt, more than any other person, is responsible for the popular acceptance of the rather revolutionary notion (until he came along) that the shortage of fiber in the digestive tracts of Westerners is responsible for a small army of civilized diseases. He discovered that primitive people, who eat much more fiber (and pass larger stools), rarely suffer from those same ills.

"I've been called the apostle of Dr. Burkitt to the Americans," says James Anderson, M.D., the University of Kentucky medical school professor whose research with diabetics—specifically the impact of high-carbohydrate, high-fiber diets on their disease—supports the British physician's theory. "I've had something to do with it here, but Dr. Burkitt was clearly the leading figure in establishing credibility for the fiber hypothesis and bringing it to the attention of the scientific community." (For more information on Dr. Anderson and his work, see pages 18-19.)

The man who accomplished this began life in 1911 as the son of a surveyor in County Fermanagh, Ireland. His early experience of medicine wasn't a positive one—a medical uncle removed his tonsils in the living room, and a surgeon took an eye injured in a rock-throwing incident. But Dr. Burkitt ended up in medicine anyway, despite starting his academic career in engineering. He gives God the credit.

"The more I prayed about it, the more I felt an overwhelming conviction that God was calling me to make this change," Dr. Burkitt once told a biographer. "It was made clear to me that medicine was what I was meant to be doing."

He made the change to medical studies in 1930, graduating from Trinity College's medical school five years later. A series of jobs followed, including a five-month stint as ship's surgeon on a freighter bound for Manchuria. He met and married his wife, Olive, served a five-year hitch as an army surgeon during World War II, and then was given the opportunity that would put him on the path to international recognition: to go to Africa as a surgeon in the Colonial Service.

Dr. Burkitt spent the next 20 years in Uganda, operating out of Mulago Hospital and its affiliated medical school in the capital city of Kampala.

A CANCER DETECTIVE

Two things happened there: He discovered the cancer, Burkitt's lymphoma, that established his reputation in the international medical community. Burkitt's lymphoma was the first cancer clearly linked to a virus, a fact that offered new hope: Many diseases of viral origin have been treated with vaccines.

And, although Dr. Burkitt returned to England in 1966, his decades in Africa provided him with the expertise and contacts he would need to develop and validate the theory that many diseases of Western civilization, including heart disease and bowel cancer, could be traced to a lack of fiber in our diet.

"In 1968, when I first became interested in the role fiber played in human health, about ten papers a year were being published on the subject," Dr. Burkitt says. "By 1980, *500* papers were being pub-

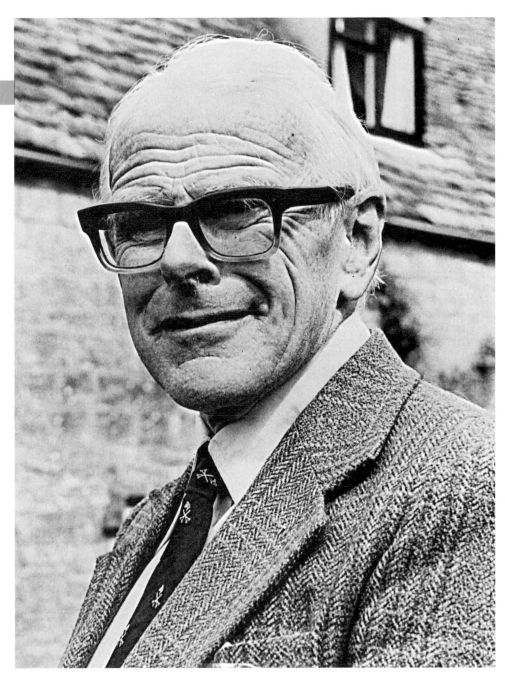

If Dr. Denis Burkitt could advise one diet change for better health, it would be to eat more brown bread. The British physician led the way in the scientific effort that established the critical importance of food fiber to human health.

lished every year. Fiber's importance is totally accepted today."

And the distinguished senior scientist is more than pleased to see people around the world changing the way they eat—adding bran to their morning cereal and deliberately selecting whole grains, beans and other high-fiber foods—as a direct result of his research, even though all the answers about how fiber works aren't in yet.

"The idea that we shouldn't do anything until everything is proved is contrary to the way we've operated throughout medical history," Dr. Burkitt says. "If you have a hypothesis that fits the facts, and it is the only one that fits the facts, and the application of which can't *possibly* do any harm and which in all probability will do enormous *good*—the only reasonable thing to do is to accept it."

Dr. Burkitt resigned his position with Britain's Medical Research Council in 1978. He resides in Gloucester but doesn't spend his days puttering in the garden. He lectures aggressively, keeping the results of his research in the public eye.

CANCER

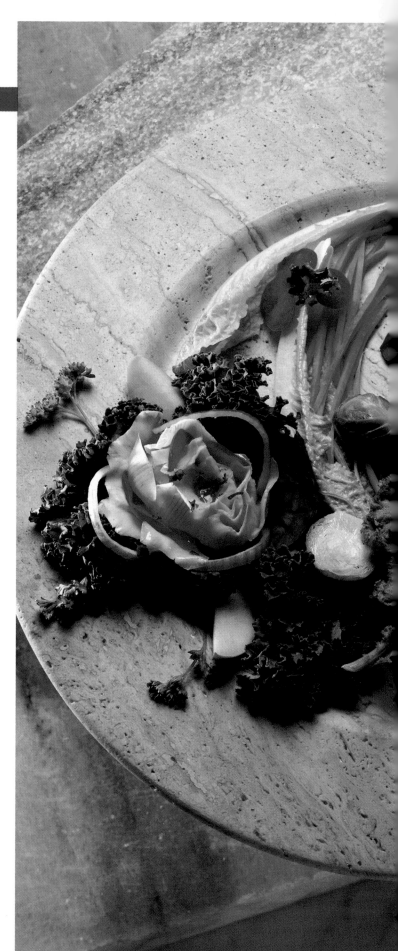

Cancer is the monster that lurks in the adult closet. And you're not the only one who lies in bed at night waiting for the door to swing open.

You've known people...You've heard the stories...Maybe you've even had the misfortune to sit holding the hand of a loved one in the last throes of the dreaded disease. You do *not* want it to happen to you and you *certainly* don't want it to touch members of your family.

You'll do anything you can to prevent cancer, including paying careful attention to diet. Yet for the past several years the popular media have overflowed with so many recommendations and counter-recommendations about which foods cause cancer and which foods prevent cancer, which things to add to your diet and which things to avoid, that the average person might well throw up his hands in despair.

If you have trouble staying on top of the latest in dietary recommendations to fight cancer, you are in august company. "It's difficult for me, too," says Daniel Nixon, M.D., associate director for cancer prevention research at the National Cancer Institute (NCI). Dr. Nixon is in charge of NCI's new Cancer and Nutrition Research Laboratory.

"Our goal is to try and make some sense out of what foods do and don't do in the cancer process," he says. He adds that he sympathizes totally with the layperson's efforts to understand the dos and don'ts of reducing the cancer risk through diet.

Yet there *are* a number of strong weapons in the great fight against cancer. A number of those weapons involve simple dietary changes.

Elaine Lanza, Ph.D., is with NCI's Division of Cancer Prevention and Control. She was responsible for the chapter on diet and cancer in the Surgeon General's report on nutrition and health, which is scheduled for release in the summer of 1988.

THE CANCER-PREVENTION DIET

Dr. Lanza says that the basic dietary recommendations (following) for preventing cancer have not changed since the National Academy of Sciences

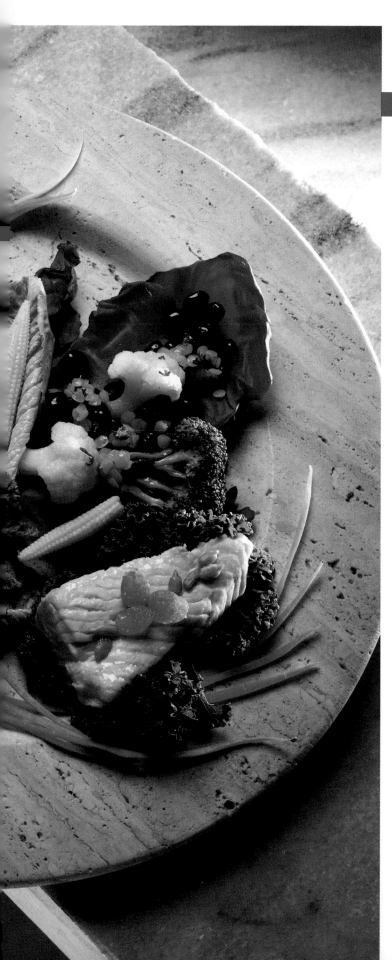

came out with them in 1982, and subsequent research supports that list with a vengeance.

- Decrease the amount of fat in your diet.
- Increase the amount of fiber in your diet.
- Avoid obesity.
- Drink alcohol in moderation, if at all.
- Minimize consumption of salt-cured, pickled and smoked foods.

Down with Fat

There has probably been more research on the role of dietary fat in developing cancer than on any other component of the diet, says Dr. Lanza. Population studies show a connection between high fat consumption and breast and colon cancer, two of the deadliest cancers in the United States in terms of sheer numbers of people who die from them.

The NCI recommends that no more than 30 percent of the calories you eat every day come from fat. Other researchers are calling for an even more drastic reduction in fat. When some of America's top cancer researchers gathered at an American Health Foundation conference to discuss the effects of fat and fiber on cancer, they determined that no more than 20 to 25 percent of dietary calories should come from fat.

Up with Fiber

The need to increase fiber in the diet is another recommendation that has been backed with solid research.

You should increase the amount of fiber in your diet to 30 grams a day, according to the NCI. To put that in perspective, Dr. Lanza says that the average American eats 10 to 12 grams of fiber a day. The NCI suggests you first attempt to reach 20 grams daily, then increase that amount to 30.

You just can't beat a salad if you're attempting to put together an anticancer meal. Just look at what this one has going for it: low in fat, high in fiber and chock-full of vitamins and minerals, even offering the special anticancer nutrients like omega-3 unsaturated fatty acids.

Decreasing the fat and increasing the fiber in your diet doesn't have to be a big deal. Just trim all the visible fat from the meat that you eat, switch to low-fat dairy products and increase your consumption of whole grains, fruits and vegetables.

Even Americans whose only vegetable is the piece of lettuce on their daily hamburger can increase their fiber intake by trading the burgers for chili a couple of times a week. The kidney beans in the chili are a good source of fiber, as are beans in general.

Look Hard at Alcohol

Just don't order a schooner of beer to go with the chili. The NCI says to "drink in moderation, if at all."

Since that recommendation was first published, researchers at the Harvard Medical School found that even three drinks a *week* put women at increased risk for breast cancer. Women who had one or more drinks a day were at 60 percent higher risk than women who did not drink.

If you are a woman who is already at high risk for developing breast cancer, you might want to take careful note of how much you drink. According to the American Cancer Society, you are at high risk if:
● You are obese.
● You have had no children or had your first pregnancy after the age of 30.
● Your mother or a sister had breast cancer.

If you men think that lets you off the hook as far as drinking is concerned, guess again. Studies on laboratory animals have established an association between heavy drinking, especially beer drinking, and cancer of the bowel.

Watch Out for Cured Foods

We have the Orient to thank for such wonderful cancer-fighting concoctions as stir fries, with their low-fat, high-fiber, high-vitamin payload.

We can also learn from Asians what *not* to eat. Those who eat a traditional diet have a high rate of stomach and esophageal cancer because they eat a lot of salt-cured, pickled and smoked foods. The

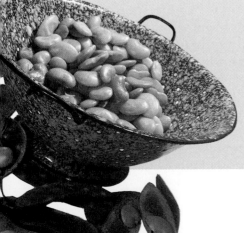

MORE CANCER FIGHTERS

Beans, rice, potatoes and seeds all contain compounds known as protease inhibitors, which may be potent cancer fighters. Try to eat some of these foods often.

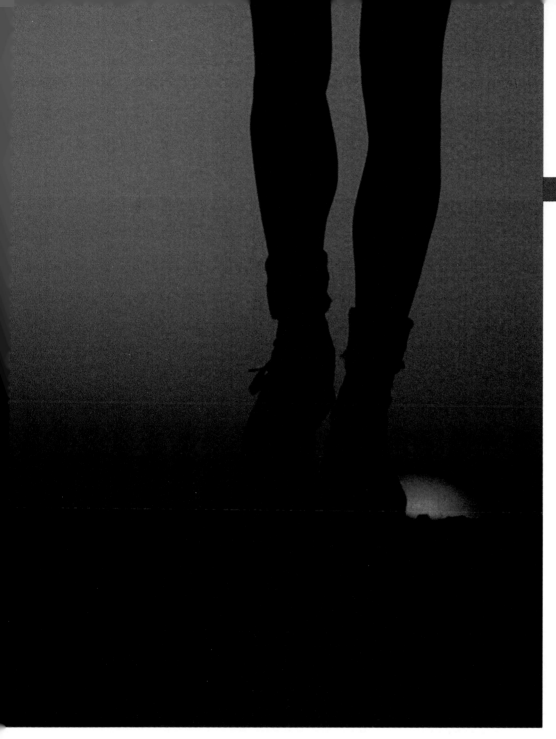

Looking beautiful is not the only reason for losing weight. People who are obese are at increased risk for certain kinds of cancers. In addition to making dietary changes, exercise. Dropping those excess pounds also may help to prevent heart disease.

high rate of stomach cancer in Japan, for example, has been traced to the large amount of smoked fish that Japanese people consume.

Even though the rate of stomach cancer is low in the United States, if you eat a lot of foods such as pickles, ham and bacon, you should cut back.

Review Your Overall Nutrition

Eating more fruits and vegetables in order to cut back on fat and increase the amount of fiber in your diet is a good bet for yet another reason. Fruits and vegetables contain all kinds of vitamins and minerals that fight cancer.

But which vitamins? Which minerals? How much is enough? Ah, there's the rub. Nobody knows. Researchers are at work all over the world studying the role of micronutrients in cancer prevention, hoping to answer just those questions. Until they do, you might want to follow the hard-boiled recommendation of one of America's top cancer researchers.

"It's advisable to eat a salad a day, a serving of a green or yellow vegetable and a fruit," says Ernst Wynder, M.D., president of the American Health Foundation.

Micronutrients currently under study include the vitamins A, C and E and the minerals calcium and selenium. According to Dr. Lanza, who is very much involved in researching micronutrients, there are probably cancer-fighting properties in fruits and vegetables that haven't even been discovered yet.

Getting enough of the "popular vitamins" doesn't have to be difficult. Lorraine Sirota, Ed.D., R.D., assistant professor of nutrition at Brooklyn College, has been involved for a few years in educating the public about reducing the dietary risk factors of cancer. She is a member of the Food and Nutrition Council of Greater New York and has conducted workshops on the subject that were supported by the American Cancer Society, New York Division.

Vitamin A. In the form of beta-carotene, it has gotten the most attention so far, says Dr. Sirota. "One large carrot a day would give a generous amount of beta-carotene." Beta-carotene is found in most fruits and vegetables that have an orange or yellow pigment, as well as in dark green, leafy vegetables.

Vitamin C. Good sources of vitamin C, she says, are citrus fruits, broccoli, cantaloupe, peppers, cauliflower, potatoes, strawberries and most dark green, leafy vegetables.

Vitamin E. It is found in whole grains, wheat germ, sunflower seeds and vegetable oils.

The main things to remember if you want to get enough vitamins and minerals are variety and freshness. "It comes down to eating more *fresh* fruits and vegetables, 'fresh' meaning less processed," says Dr. Sirota. "We're not talking about Mom's apple pie and canned peaches in syrup."

Cruciferous vegetables. When you select fresh vegetables, be sure to include members of the cruciferous family. Since 1982 the American Cancer Society has recommended eating cruciferous vegetables on a regular basis. These vegetables contain certain chemical substances that, in animal studies, play a role in preventing or reducing the risk of cancer. Cruciferous vegetables include broccoli, cabbage, mustard greens, cauliflower, rutabagas, turnips and brussels sprouts. But don't overload on just this one family of vegetables to the exclusion of all others. The way to go here is to include small serv-ings of cruciferous vegetables in your diet on a regular basis, perhaps in a salad.

Fish oil. Is there no end to the claims for omega-3 oils found in such abundance in mackerel, salmon, herring, tuna and other fish? Now a study on lab animals has shown that these oils can slow the growth of cancerous tumors. Another lab study showed that cancer in animals fed these fish oils spread less frequently to other parts of the body. So substitute fish for meat a couple of times a week, and you'll be cutting back on saturated fat while increasing your omega-3.

Check Your Cooking Methods

Finally, a word about cooking. Be cautious about browning meats. John Weisburger, M.D., Ph.D., a senior member of the American Health Foundation, says he has been doing research based on a 1977 Japanese study that concluded that browning foods produces cancer-causing chemicals. The browning process does indeed create powerful carcinogens, but whether they are produced in sufficient amounts to be of concern has not yet been determined.

In the meantime, to be on the safe side, you might want to add 10 percent soy protein to your hamburgers, says Dr. Weisburger. The soy protein helps to lower the formation of the carcinogens on the surface of the meat while also lowering your fat intake. Dr. Weisburger says he would like to see school systems across the country routinely add soy protein to hamburgers for precisely this reason.

You might also use your microwave oven more often, as it uses a cooking method that does not involve browning. If you eat less red meat and throw away the skin from poultry (both ploys to reduce your fat intake), you will also reduce your intake of these chemicals.

From the recommendation to reduce fat to the less common suggestion to use soy protein—all of the advice is good, and none will do harm. Incorporate these helpful recommendations into your daily living to help keep that malignant monster trapped in his dark closet.

CANCER
A DAY OF INTENSIVE HEALING

A.M.	NOON	P.M.

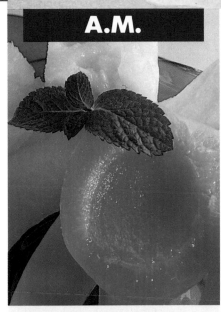 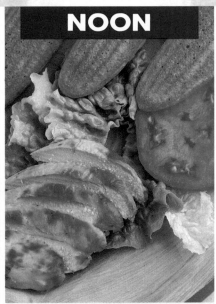 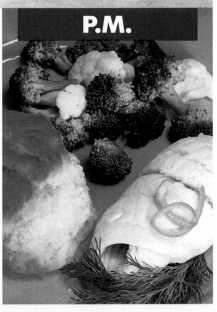

A.M.

Apricot nectar
Oat bran cereal
Low-fat pumpkin muffin
Fruit cup (chunk pineapple, papaya and mango)

NOON

Beans 'n' greens soup (soybeans, navy beans, kale and spinach)
Sliced chicken breast, tomato and lettuce on whole wheat bread
Cornbread sticks
Cantaloupe chunks and berries
Skim milk

P.M.

Red cabbage and onion slaw with horseradish sauce
Citrus-marinated flounder
Candied sweet potatoes
Steamed broccoli and cauliflower
Oatmeal-buttermilk biscuits
Strawberries and yogurt

DISASTER PLATE

Grilled hot dog with cheese, wrapped in bacon
Hot dog roll
Potato chips
Vanilla shake

Looking for a good cancer-fighting meal? Look elsewhere. The grilled hot

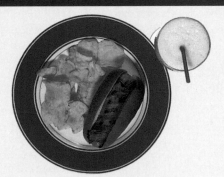

dog has a number of counts against it. Cured meat contains nitrates. This cured meat is wrapped in *more* cured meat, then cooked using a method that may create even more carcinogens. The cheese, chips and shake are fatty and virtually fiberless.

INTENSIVE HEALING RECIPES: CANCER

Some nutrients may help provide significant protection against cancer. Among them are beta-carotene, calcium and vitamin C, all of which are found in these recipes. Serve Vegetable Lo Mein as a tasty, healthful, change-of-pace main dish and Warm Squash Salad in Cabbage Cups as a colorful addition to any meal.

WARM SQUASH SALAD IN CABBAGE CUPS

½ lb. crookneck squash (neck pumpkin), peeled and cut into julienne strips
2 tomatoes, cut into chunks
⅓ cup broccoli stems, peeled and cut into julienne strips
1 leek, topped and cut into julienne strips
3 Tbsp. buttermilk
½ tsp. Dijon-style mustard
2 tsp. finely minced fresh basil
 Pinch of curry powder
4 purple or green cabbage leaves
 Sprigs of basil, for garnish

In a medium-size saucepan, steam squash until tender, about 12 minutes or more.

In a large bowl, combine squash, tomatoes, broccoli and leeks.

In a small bowl, whisk buttermilk, mustard, basil and curry powder. Pour over squash mixture and toss well to combine.

Place cabbage leaves on a serving platter. Spoon squash mixture onto leaves, garnish with basil sprigs and serve warm.

Yield: 4 servings

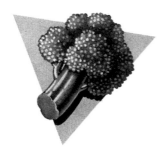

A fatty diet is related to several types of cancer. You won't find any significant fat in broccoli. What you *will* find is lots of vitamin C, vitamin A and fiber.

VEGETABLE LO MEIN

1 Tbsp. peanut oil
1 medium-size onion, sliced into 12 wedges
2 carrots, cut into julienne strips
1 large sweet red pepper, cut into julienne strips
1 cup broccoli florets, cut into bite-size pieces
1 large clove garlic, thinly sliced
2 Tbsp. Chinese oyster sauce
1 Tbsp. mirin*
2 cups cooked spaghetti or vermicelli
 Splash of toasted sesame oil, or to taste

Heat a large wok, then add peanut oil. Add onions and stir-fry until slightly tender and beginning to be spotted with brown, about 2 minutes. Add carrots, peppers, broccoli and garlic and continue to stir-fry for about 2 minutes.

In a small bowl, stir together oyster sauce and mirin. Pour over vegetables, immediately add spaghetti or vermicelli and toss well to combine.

Remove from heat, splash with sesame oil, toss lightly and serve hot.

Yield: 4 servings

*Mirin is a sweet rice vinegar and is available at oriental markets.

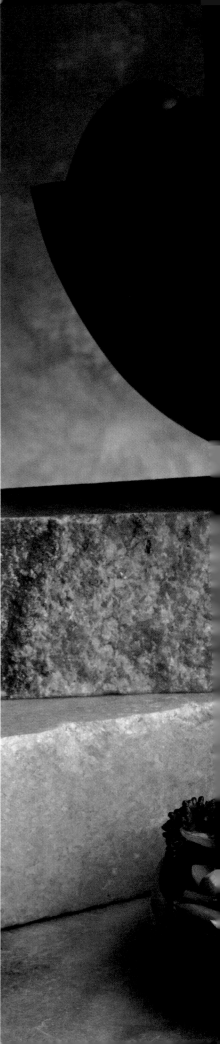

34

Vegetable Lo Mein

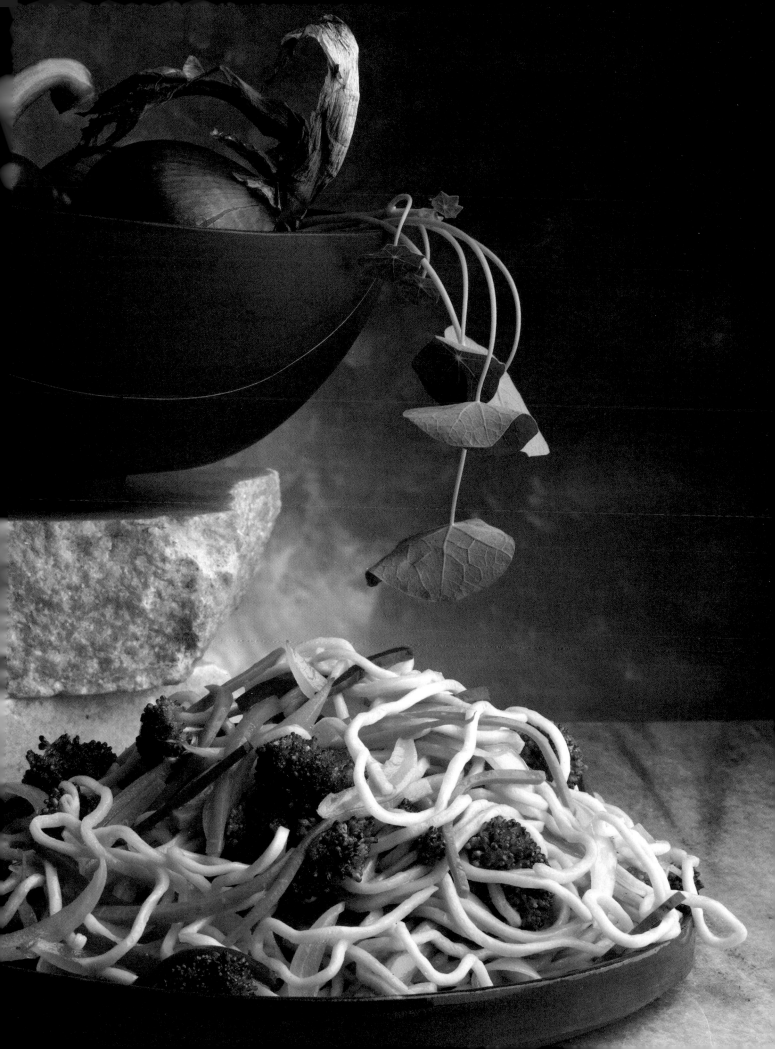

CELIAC DISEASE

You can eat popcorn and corn chips but not pretzels. You can eat corn bread, potato rolls and rice cakes but not white bread, whole wheat or rye. You can eat homemade soup but not canned, roast chicken but not processed, cheese but not cheese spreads.

What's the common denominator behind such an oddball list? It's the absence or presence of gluten—a protein found in wheat, oats, rye and barley. If you have celiac disease, it hits your gut like a bomb. It flattens all of the normally erect intestinal structures that digest and absorb your food, and it leaves you, as one gastroenterologist said, "starving in the midst of plenty."

You can avoid wasting away into nothingness by following a gluten-free diet, says Henry J. Binder, M.D., a gastroenterologist at Yale University. But that's not always easy, he adds, because gluten is frequently hidden in even the most common foods.

"You have to go through your supermarket with a book in your hand," agrees Richard McCallum, M.D., who is chairman of the Department of Gastroenterology at the University of Virginia Medical School. Gluten can be tucked away in chocolate milk, dumplings, meat patties, whipped cream substitutes, salad dressings, packaged pudding mixes, dry-roasted nuts, the cream sauces or breading on frozen foods and the barbecue seasoning on corn chips or potato chips (which are otherwise okay). It's in Worcestershire sauce, baked beans, even the wafers your church uses for Communion and, occasionally, instant coffee.

Looking for hidden gluten can be exhausting. An alternative is to get out your mixing bowls and make all your meals from scratch.

COOKING WITHOUT WHEAT

Grandma's recipe for dumplings calls for regular wheat flour—and so do most recipes in most cookbooks. Even so, those with celiac disease can cook and bake their favorites by substituting an acceptable flour for the wheat. (Use the guide at right to determine the proper amount.)

Stick to potato, rice, soy or tapioca flours if you're sensitive to gluten. Potato and soy flours are best used in combination with the other two.

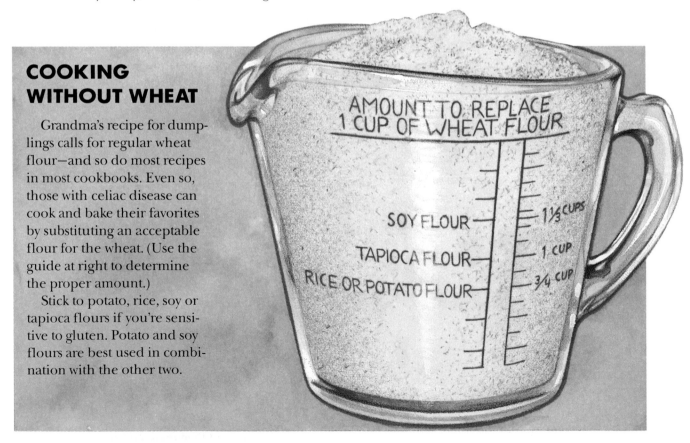

AMOUNT TO REPLACE 1 CUP OF WHEAT FLOUR

SOY FLOUR — 1⅓ CUPS
TAPIOCA FLOUR — 1 CUP
RICE OR POTATO FLOUR — ¾ CUP

INTENSIVE HEALING RECIPES:
CELIAC DISEASE

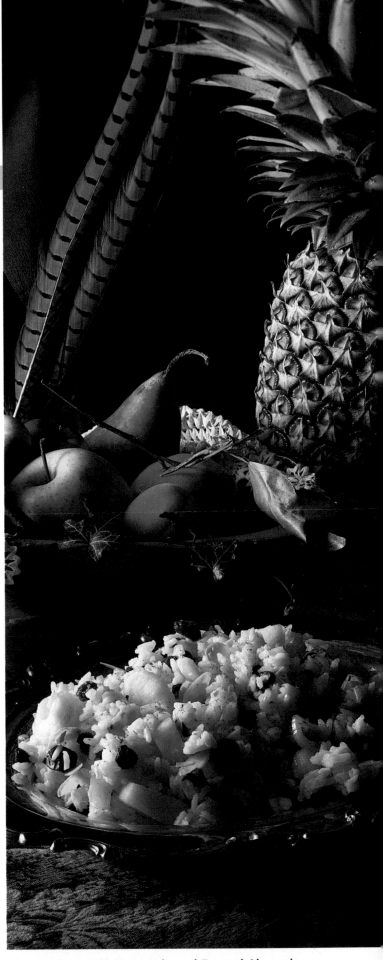

These recipes are just two examples of the versatility of rice, a gluten-free grain.

RICE STUFFING WITH PINEAPPLE AND TOASTED ALMONDS

2½ cups cooked rice
1   cup chopped pineapple
2   shallots, finely minced
½   cup raisins
⅓   cup chopped toasted almonds
¼   tsp. freshly ground allspice

Combine all ingredients in a medium-size bowl. Use to stuff a whole chicken, fish fillets, chicken breasts, Cornish hens or vegetables such as sweet peppers or large onions.

Yield: 6 servings (enough to stuff a 4-pound chicken or 6 large fish fillets)

RICE CRUST FOR SAVORY OR SWEET PIES

1   egg
1   egg white
3   cups cooked rice

Preheat the oven to 350°F.
   In a medium-size bowl, whisk egg and egg white until they change color to a clear, bright yellow,

about 30 to 45 seconds. Then add rice and combine well.
   Spray a 9 × 2-inch glass pie plate with nonstick spray. Place rice mixture in pie plate and, using a piece of waxed paper and your hand, flatten mixture into a firm crust. Make sure to extend it up the sides of the pie plate.
   Bake until crust is dry to the touch and clicks when tapped with a fingernail, about 20 to 25 minutes.
   Fill crust with pudding or mousse and chill until set. Or fill with quiche-type mixture and continue to bake until set, about 40 minutes.

Yield: one 9-inch crust

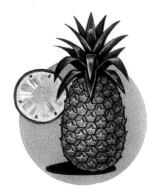

This tropical treat packs a lot of nutrition. One slice of fresh pineapple will give you vitamin C, fiber and calcium.

Rice Stuffing with Pineapple and Toasted Almonds

CHOLESTEROL

Cholesterol. Not since Hollywood sent us The Blob has a yukky fatlike substance received so much publicity or given rise to so much fear.

In part, the fear is well deserved. Numerous studies show that the more little blobs of cholesterol you have meandering through your blood, the greater your risk of suffering a heart attack—America's biggest killer.

Look at the illustrations on this page. Here's how cholesterol, along with other errant substances like triglycerides, can form a waxy plaque that sticks to your artery walls. When the plaque grows and starts to restrict the passage of blood, we call this condition atherosclerosis or, more commonly, hardened arteries. When the artery becomes severely narrowed or entirely blocked, and blood (on which the heart depends for essential oxygen) can no longer pass, tragedy occurs.

The amount of cholesterol in your blood is typically measured in milligrams per deciliter. The National Heart, Lung, and Blood Institute (NHLBI) and the American Heart Association (AHA) say that as long as you have less than 200 milligrams of cholesterol per deciliter of blood (commonly expressed as 200 mg/dl), you're relatively safe. Over 200, they say, and you're running a risk. Sadly—because cholesterol can largely be controlled—more than half of all adult Americans are estimated to fall into the latter, daredevilish group.

A STRONG LINK TO DIET

How you might have gotten yourself into the elevated risk group is the key to getting yourself out: your food choices. "Diet is one of the major causes of high cholesterol," says Scott Grundy, M.D., Ph.D., director of the Center for Human Nutrition at the University of Texas Health Science Center. "Therefore, dietary therapy should be the first part of treatment."

Before you mount your forces against cholesterol, logic dictates that you first know whether yours is too high. Have you had your blood tested yet? The AHA strongly recommends that if you're age 20 or older, you do so.

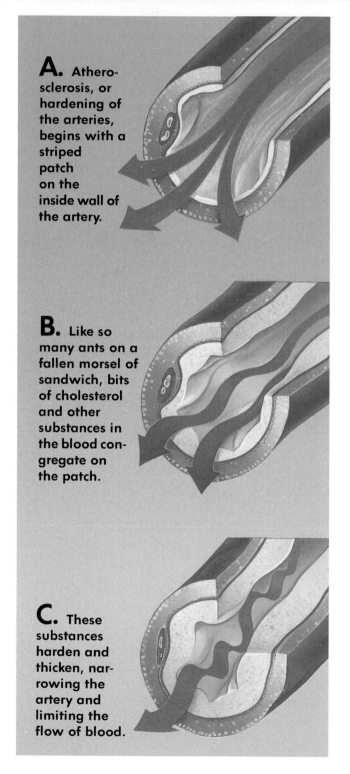

A. Atherosclerosis, or hardening of the arteries, begins with a striped patch on the inside wall of the artery.

B. Like so many ants on a fallen morsel of sandwich, bits of cholesterol and other substances in the blood congregate on the patch.

C. These substances harden and thicken, narrowing the artery and limiting the flow of blood.

HDL AND LDL CHOLESTEROL—THE GOOD, THE BAD AND THE UGLY

Cholesterol comes in several kinds of packages. Most notably, there's one variety called high-density lipoprotein, or HDL, cholesterol and another larger package called low-density lipoprotein, or LDL, cholesterol. They are related, but—like Patty and Cathy on the old "Patty Duke Show"—they're as different as two cousins can be.

The LDLs are primarily a mixture of cholesterol and protein that the blood carries to all parts of the body. The body needs some cholesterol for its everyday functions like producing hormones and digestive acids. What the body needs, it makes for itself—any extra you get from a fatty diet becomes surplus. Since this surplus, which can become dangerous plaque, travels through the body as LDL cholesterol, it is often called the bad cholesterol.

HDL cholesterol, on the other hand, is often called the good cholesterol. This is because it picks up the excess cholesterol and heads to the liver, taking trouble with it. In the liver, the cholesterol is reprocessed or removed from the body.

After you've taken a blood test to measure your cholesterol, you'll be given figures for your LDL cholesterol level, your HDL cholesterol level and your total cholesterol level. Keeping in mind that LDL is bad and HDL good, you're shooting for a low LDL number and a high HDL number.

According to NHLBI guidelines, your LDL level should be *below* 130 mg/dl; your HDL level should be *above* 35 mg/dl and your total cholesterol level should be *below* 200 mg/dl.

Ah . . . perhaps you're thinking about a friend who has had such a test, and how the printout of the results came heavily peppered with acronyms like LDL and HDL—sounding as complex as an exercise in an advanced trigonometry textbook. But it's really not that complicated. All you'll need to know is explained in the accompanying box.

Let's assume you've already had your blood tested and you've learned that your cholesterol level is 220 mg/dl. This puts you, according to the NHLBI, in the "borderline-high" range. Don't panic!

The first thing to do: Check it again. Cholesterol testing is tricky business. The AHA suggests that before you start to fret, have at least a second test done. Average the two scores. (We'll assume, again, that you're still in the borderline-high range.)

Now what?

Obviously, the first thing you do is run right to your refrigerator, swing open the door, plunk those eggs one by one down the garbage disposal and swear by all that's holy that you'll never ever eat cholesterol again . . . . Right?

Not exactly.

The difference between *dietary* cholesterol and *blood* cholesterol is a point of great confusion for many people, says John LaRosa, M.D., dean of clinical affairs for George Washington University and chairman of the AHA's Nutrition Committee. "Dietary cholesterol is *not* the most important determinant of cholesterol levels in the blood—*saturated fat* is the larger culprit," he says.

Foods high in cholesterol and foods high in saturated fat will both tend to raise your blood cholesterol level. As chance would have it, those foods high in cholesterol are usually (but not always) also high in saturated fat, and vice-versa. This is most fortunate, for it makes anticholesterol diet planning a lot easier.

THE ART OF SMART EATING

Whether you're in the borderline-high cholesterol range (as we previously assumed you are) or in the high range (generally considered 240 mg/dl or above), changes in diet alone should be enough to snip your cholesterol down to a respectable level.

To develop your new anticholesterol diet, you'll need to learn to identify those foods high in saturated fat and cholesterol. "Identifying foods high in cholesterol is relatively easy," says Peter Wilson, M.D., director of laboratories at the Framingham Heart

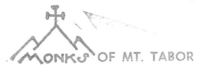

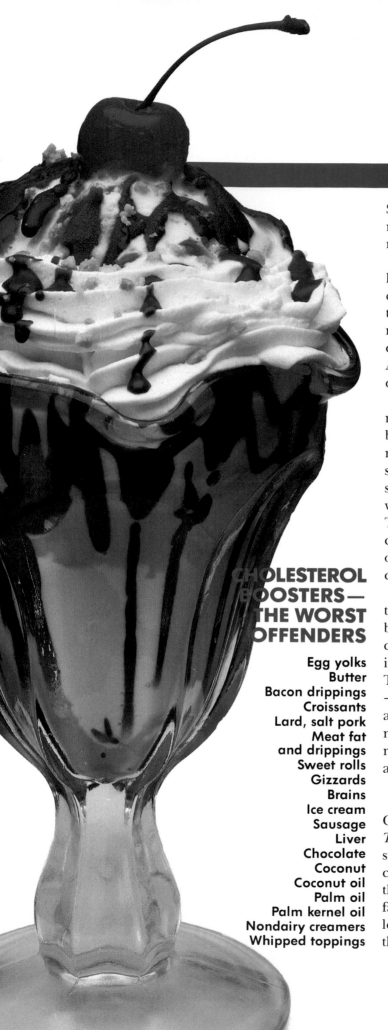

CHOLESTEROL
BOOSTERS—
THE WORST
OFFENDERS

Egg yolks
Butter
Bacon drippings
Croissants
Lard, salt pork
Meat fat
and drippings
Sweet rolls
Gizzards
Brains
Ice cream
Sausage
Liver
Chocolate
Coconut
Coconut oil
Palm oil
Palm kernel oil
Nondairy creamers
Whipped toppings

Study (one of the oldest and most extensive heart research projects in the world). "There aren't that many, and they are mostly animal products."

Egg yolks, says Dr. Wilson, are the first thing to keep an eye out for. (Egg whites are fine.) One yolk contains about 270 milligrams of cholesterol, nearly the government's recommended daily limit of 300 milligrams. Look out for all products made with eggs, such as many baked goods, says Dr. Wilson. Also beware of cholesterol-packed organ meats. And don't gorge yourself on dairy products, either.

As for saturated fats, Dr. Wilson says it's easier to run into trouble with them, as they can be found in both the plant and animal kingdoms. One clue to recognizing a saturated fat, says Dr. Wilson, is that it solidifies at room temperature. Foods sky-high in saturated fat—and worthy of caution—include butter, whole milk, cream, ice cream, cheese and fatty meats. Three plant oils to avoid, all commonly used in processed foods (many of which herald "no cholesterol!!" on the label), are palm oil, palm kernel oil and coconut oil.

You're going to want to know both the cholesterol *and* the saturated fat content of a given food before deciding whether it belongs in your anti-cholesterol diet. Again, many foods that are high in one are high in the other, but there are exceptions. The three tropical plant oils are important exceptions —they contain no cholesterol. Certain shellfish, such as shrimp and lobster, are exceptions as well—they're reasonably high in cholesterol but very low in saturated fat. (Other shellfish, like clams and mussels, aren't as high in cholesterol.)

So, do we eat shrimp and lobster or not?

Eat 'em, say William Connor, M.D., and Sonja Connor, a registered dietitian, who are authors of *The New American Diet.* The Connors developed a system for rating various foods based on both their cholesterol and saturated fat contents. They call it the CSI index. Shellfish, because they're so low in fat, turn out to be a better choice than even the leanest red meat. (For more on the CSI index, see the box "Rating the Fats" on pages 82–83.) All the same, the AHA suggests that if you like shrimp and lobster, eat them only in moderation.

FINE-TUNING YOUR LEVEL

There's little doubt in the medical community that—besides heredity—two key determinants of your blood cholesterol level are those already mentioned: saturated fat and dietary cholesterol. But recent studies suggest that other factors may be quite important as well.

Cut total calories; stay thin. Tubbiness can increase your blood cholesterol level. "Caloric intake and obesity are important factors," says Dr. LaRosa. A fat person will tend to produce more low-density lipoprotein (LDL) cholesterol—the bad kind of blood cholesterol—than will a thin person, he explains.

Be active. Exercise may help you increase your level of high-density lipoprotein (HDL) cholesterol —the good kind of blood cholesterol. It may also help protect against obesity and high blood pressure—two other risk factors for coronary heart disease.

Eat less total fat. Most Americans take in 35 to 40 percent of their calories from fat. The NHLBI's National Cholesterol Education Program suggests you don't go above 30 percent. Reduced fat intake will help you in two ways: It will help you cut down on saturated fat and will help you lose weight.

Choose your fats wisely. The worst kind of fat is saturated fat. So when it is replaced in the diet by other fats—monounsaturated or polyunsaturated—blood cholesterol is reduced. Dr. Wilson suggests that when fat is eaten at all, it be either monounsaturated or polyunsaturated at least two-thirds of the time.

Polyunsaturated fats include safflower, sunflower, corn and soybean oils. Monounsaturated fats include olive, canola and peanut oils. Oils can be used for spreading (in the form of margarine), for cooking, instead of butter or lard, or on salads.

There is some evidence to suggest that monounsaturated fats may be a better choice than polyunsaturates, says Dr. LaRosa. They not only lower the level of LDL, the dangerous cholesterol, but

HDL: A NICE, HEALTHY BONUS

It's called the good cholesterol, but just how good is HDL cholesterol?

One study, as illustrated here, shows that your level of HDL cholesterol (on the horizontal line) can greatly affect your risk of coronary heart disease.

Most experts, however, say that maintaining a low level of LDL cholesterol should be your top priority. Having a good level of HDL cholesterol should be considered a nice, healthy bonus.

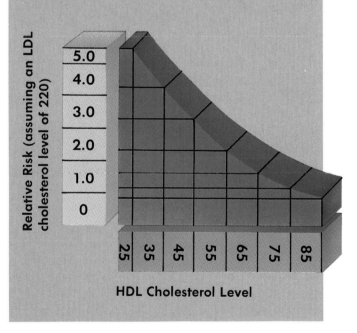

HDL Cholesterol Level

seem to leave the level of HDL, the good cholesterol, where it is.

GOING ON THE OFFENSIVE

Experts with NHLBI say that once you've begun your anticholesterol diet, your cholesterol level should drop somewhat within two to three weeks. How much it drops, and how fast, will depend on the amount of saturated fat in your diet to begin with, your blood cholesterol level prior to starting the diet, how well you follow your new diet and your own metabolism.

Let's assume you've been on an anticholesterol diet for several months now and you've successfully lowered your blood cholesterol from 220 to 180. What next? First, give yourself a hearty pat on the back. Dr. Wilson says that for those with elevated blood cholesterol levels, every 1 percent drop can mean a 2 percent reduction in the risk of a heart attack. So if you maintain your diet, you can substantially reduce your risk—by as much as 80 percent.

You now want to stabilize your cholesterol level. But does that mean you can never again eat scrambled eggs for breakfast?

Not necessarily. One study reported in the *British Medical Journal* set out to answer just that question. The researchers concluded that a few eggs a week shouldn't set you back—as long as your diet contin-

ues to be low in saturated fat and otherwise healthy.

Otherwise healthy? Aside from those blubbery foods that you want to exclude from your diet, there are several foods you may want to *include*.

Feed yourself fish. Fish may be an excellent way of tackling high cholesterol. Some scientists believe it explains a bizarre paradox: that Greenland Eskimos eat large amounts of animal fats such as seal meat and whale blubber yet have very low rates of heart disease. (They also eat a lot of fish.)

Fish oil contains a special kind of polyunsaturated fat called omega-3. In the entry on triglycerides beginning on page 156, you'll read about omega-3's proven ability to reduce the level of triglycerides in the blood. As for fish oil's powers over cholesterol, the evidence is also impressive.

Some researchers say omega-3 (often sold in supplement form as EPA or DHA) can, in effect, grease certain blood cells, making them less likely to snag the blood vessel wall and clot. Others say it can

CHOLESTEROL BUSTERS

To beat high cholesterol, you'll need to cut down on saturated fat and cholesterol in your diet. But at the same time, adding certain foods to your diet may be tremendously helpful. In a study done in India, heart patients fed garlic daily showed significant decreases in cholesterol after eight months. Onions, too, appear to share

some of garlic's cholesterol-fighting punch.

Another study found that men placed on an avocado-rich diet experienced cholesterol drops of between 9 and 43 percent. And the most highly touted cholesterol busters of all may be fish and certain fibers, such as pectin and oat bran.

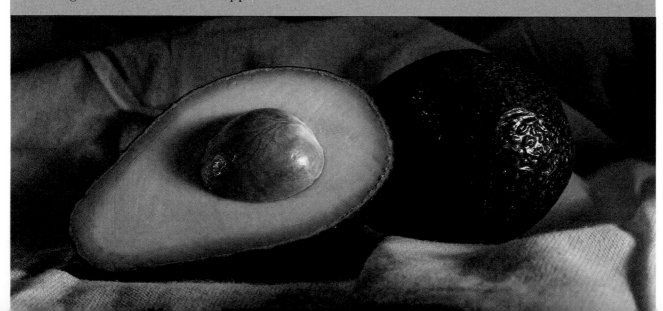

lower the level of LDL and raise the level of HDL. Researchers at the University of Chicago Medical Center say their studies on animals prove fish oil inhibits the formation of plaque buildup on artery walls—even when gobs of cholesterol are present in the blood. "Fish oil works at the vessel wall level to counteract the effects of a high-cholesterol diet," says Dragoslava Vesselinovitch, D.V.M., associate professor of pathology.

Dr. Vesselinovitch and her physician colleagues advise eating fish three times a week. The best fish are the deep-water, rich-in-oil varieties, like mackerel, bluefish and salmon. "But any fish is good," says Dr. Vesselinovitch.

While fish is good food in just about anyone's book, neither the researchers from the University of Chicago, the NHLBI nor the AHA would advocate the use of fish-oil capsules. Research hasn't shown exactly how much of the fish oil you need to get the beneficial effects.

Choose fiber, but choose well. Dietary fiber is generally accepted as a cholesterol-fighting champ. "But," says David Kritchevsky, M.D., associate director of Philadelphia's Wistar Institute, "that's not to say all fiber is useful—insoluble fiber such as bran is virtually useless in reducing cholesterol." It's the *soluble* fibers, such as pectin and oat gum (which occurs in oat bran), which can cut your cholesterol level down to size, he says.

Researchers with the U.S. Department of Agriculture have investigated how these fibers work their magic. It's a complicated affair involving the binding of certain digestive acids, but what it all boils down to is a simple equation: Your cholesterol level may be lowered "10 to 20 percent just by eating two carrots a day," say the researchers. Two other pectin-rich vegetables, cabbage and broccoli, may be just as useful, they add.

Oat bran, available in specialty food stores and some supermarkets, has been shown to be just as effective as pectin. And it doesn't take much. In one study, men were able to lower their cholesterol by 8.5 percent in six weeks by adding to their diet

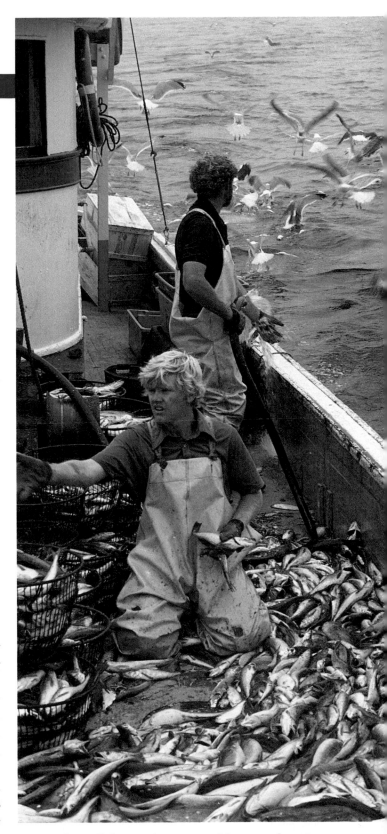

Eating these fish may be as good for your heart as the exercise involved in netting them.

only 2 ounces of oat bran a day, in the form of oat-bran muffins.

A LIFELONG PLAN

The more you learn about cholesterol, the more you'll learn about the controversies. Exactly where the ideal cholesterol level falls for a typical adult over age 40 is one item of debate. Dr. Kritchevsky says you should keep your cholesterol level below 240 mg/dl or so. S. Boyd Eaton, M.D., of Emory University, advocate of the "Stone Age Diet" (see page 74), urges you to limit your level to 160. He keeps his own at 130. Smack in the middle, advocating 200 mg/dl, are the NHLBI, the AHA and, probably, most doctors. There is general agreement, however, that the more you reduce your level, the more you reduce your risk of heart attack.

A lifelong cholesterol-reduction diet should be accompanied by regular checkups. A blood test every five years or less for those with desirable levels of blood cholesterol is recommended by the NHLBI. For those in the borderline-high range (200 to 239 mg/dl), yearly testing is recommended. For anyone with a level of 240 or higher, medical supervision is advised. Working with a physician is also advised for those in the borderline range with other risk factors, such as high blood pressure or a smoking habit.

If you come under a doctor's care for high cholesterol, you may be treated with one of a number of drugs. *All* of these drugs are administered to complement dietary therapy. They are never substitutes for eating wisely and leanly.

Whatever you stand to gain by eating a diet low in fat and cholesterol—and it certainly seems substantial—the costs are relatively small. After all, with an enormous menu of fish, fruits, vegetables, beans, grains, lean meat and low-fat dairy products to choose from, how tough is it going to be to limit those greasy-spoon specials?

WHERE'S THE PECTIN?

It's easy to add more cholesterol-lowering pectin to your diet. By doing so, you'll find yourself eating foods rich in fiber, vitamins and minerals and low in fat and calories. The table below lists some of the top pectin choices.

FOOD	PORTION	PECTIN (G)	FOOD	PORTION	PECTIN (G)
Soybeans, mature, dried, cooked	1 cup	2.60	Hazelnuts, dried, raw	1 oz.	0.85
Figs, dried, with skin	5	2.26	Lima beans, boiled	½ cup	0.85
Orange	1 med.	2.21	Carrot	1	0.78
Chestnuts, dried	1 oz.	2.10	Pistachios, dried	1 oz.	0.77
Pear	1 med.	1.83	Peanuts, dried	1 oz.	0.74
Potato	1 med.	1.79	Peach	1 med.	0.70
Sweet potato, boiled, mashed	½ cup	1.31	Peas, boiled	½ cup	0.64
Brussels sprouts, frozen, boiled	½ cup	1.09	Almonds, dried	1 oz.	0.62
Apple	1 med.	1.08	Walnuts, dried	1 oz.	0.57
Papaya	½	1.06	Green beans, frozen, boiled	½ cup	0.50
Broccoli spears, frozen, boiled	½ cup	0.97	Lemon	1	0.46
Banana	1 med.	0.91	Summer squash, boiled	½ cup	0.45
Strawberries	1 cup	0.89	Grapefruit	½ med.	0.29
Tomato	1 med.	0.86	Spinach, raw, chopped	½ cup	0.22

CHOLESTEROL
A DAY OF INTENSIVE HEALING

A.M.	NOON	P.M.

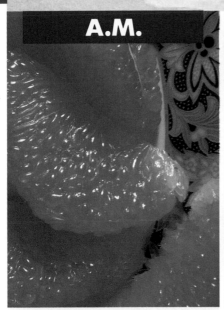
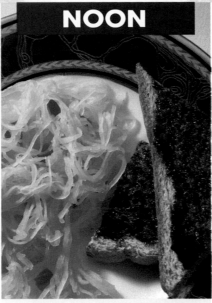
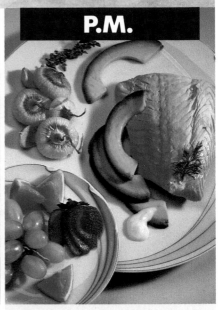

Grapefruit half
Oat bran cereal with raisins and skim milk
Applesauce with cinnamon
Hot tea with lemon

Five-bean and barley soup
Confetti spaghetti squash with peppers, onions and garlic
Cracked wheat bread with apple butter
Chopped figs and banana slices
Sparkling water and apple juice

Avocado slices with nonfat yogurt
Poached salmon
Brown rice pilaf with lentils
Oven-roasted onions and garlic with thyme
Orange wedges, strawberries and green grapes

DISASTER PLATE

Eggs Benedict (eggs, sauce and ham)
Croissant with butter
Coffee with cream

Want to send your cholesterol level into orbit? Have some eggs Benedict (each yolk is filthy rich

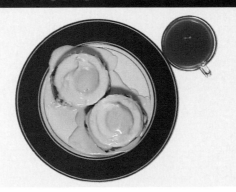

in cholesterol, and ham and hollandaise sauce add even more), a croissant with butter (great for scooping up any remaining yolk) and super-light coffee (pass the cream—or non-dairy creamer made with saturated coconut oil).

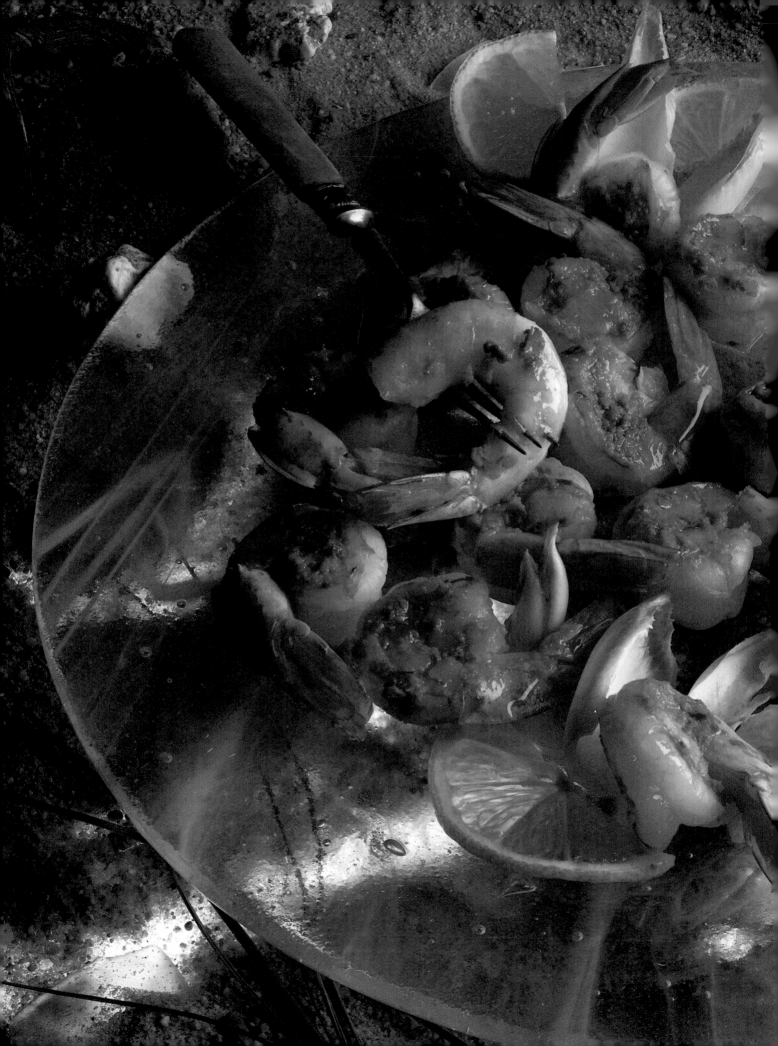

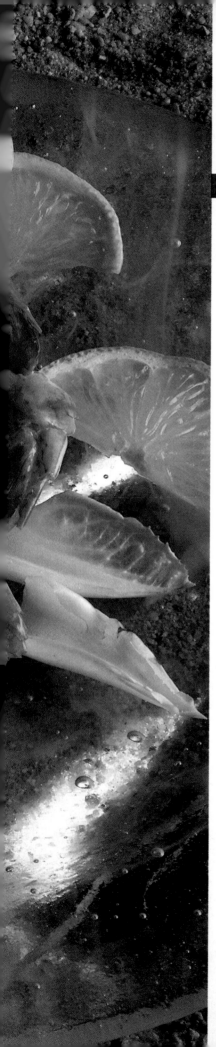

INTENSIVE HEALING RECIPES:
CHOLESTEROL

These recipes present several appetizing ways to fight cholesterol. They are low in harmful fats and are made with ingredients that are proven cholesterol fighters. The omega-3 fatty acids in fish and the fiber in oats and oat bran, as well as garlic and onions, have all been shown to promote cholesterol reduction.

CHILLED SHRIMP WITH GREEN OLIVES AND SAFFRON

1	lb. large shrimp, peeled and deveined
⅓	tsp. saffron threads, crushed
	Juice and pulp of ½ lemon
7	tiny pitted green olives
1	small clove garlic
1	tsp. olive oil

In a large saucepan, simmer shrimp in boiling water until opaque and just cooked through, about 3½ to 4 minutes.

Meanwhile, in a small saucepan, heat saffron and lemon juice and pulp until fragrant, about 30 seconds. (You can also do this in a microwave. Place saffron and lemon in a microwave-safe dish, cover and microwave on full power for about 15 seconds.)

With a mortar and pestle or spice grinder, mash olives, garlic and oil until a smooth paste forms. Then stir in saffron mixture.

When shrimp are cooked, drain and pat dry. Place in a medium-size Pyrex bowl, along with olive mixture. Marinate for about 2 hours in the refrigerator. Serve cold with crusty bread or endive leaves.

Yield: 4 servings

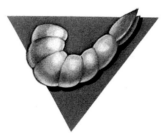

Shrimp may have some cholesterol, but it also has a good amount of omega-3 fatty acids — known cholesterol fighters.

FLOUNDER WITH MUSTARD AND THYME

1	lb. flounder fillets
¼	cup oat bran
2	tsp. olive oil
½	cup chicken stock
1	tsp. Dijon mustard
½	tsp. dried thyme
	Fresh thyme sprigs or lemon slices, for garnish

Coat fillets with oat bran.

Heat oil in a nonstick skillet. Add fillets and sauté until cooked through, about 3½ minutes on each side.

Carefully remove fish to a heated platter. Pour stock into the skillet and whisk in mustard and thyme. Bring to a boil and continue to boil until reduced by half. Pour over fish and serve hot, garnished with thyme sprigs or lemon slices.

Yield: 4 servings

FRESH SALMON WITH GARLIC AND CORIANDER

2	tsp. olive oil
1	lb. salmon fillets, skin removed
2	cloves garlic, finely minced
1	Tbsp. minced fresh coriander
	Splash of hot pepper sauce, or to taste
	Juice and pulp of 1 lime

Chilled Shrimp with Green Olives and Saffron

Juice and pulp of
1 lemon
Minced scallions
and tomato slices,
for garnish

Heat a nonstick skillet over medium-high heat, then add oil. When oil is warm, add fillets and sauté for 4 or 5 minutes on each side, until just about cooked through. Handle salmon gently to keep pieces whole.

Add garlic, coriander, hot pepper sauce, lime and lemon to the skillet and cook for about 1 minute. Do not allow coriander to turn brown.

Remove fillets from skillet and refrigerate, covered, until chilled. To serve, place on a serving platter, sprinkle with scallions and add tomato slices.

Yield: 4 servings

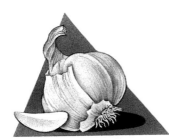

Garlic may lower levels of cholesterol in the blood. One study showed that frequent garlic eaters had levels 23 percent lower than those that ate none.

POACHED CHICKEN WITH CHINESE VINAIGRETTE

1   tsp. minced peeled ginger root
2   cloves garlic, crushed
1   lb. chicken cutlets
1   green pepper, cut into julienne strips
2   scallions, cut into julienne strips
2   Tbsp. rice vinegar
1   tsp. toasted sesame oil
2   tsp. hoisin sauce
    Red and green lettuce leaves

In a large skillet, place enough water to cover chicken and bring to a simmer over medium heat. Add ginger, garlic and chicken, then cover and poach until chicken is cooked through, about 10 to 15 minutes, depending on thickness. Drain chicken and place in the refrigerator to chill.

When chicken is thoroughly chilled, shred it with your fingers, then place in a medium-size bowl. Add peppers and scallions and set aside.

In a small bowl, whisk vinegar, oil and hoisin. Pour mixture over chicken and toss well until all pieces are coated.

To serve, mound chicken on a serving platter.

Scoop onto a lettuce leaf, roll and eat.

Yield: 4 servings

TUNA STEAKS WITH OLIVE OIL AND THYME

1   lb. fresh tuna (4 pieces)
1   tsp. dried thyme
1   Tbsp. plus 1 tsp. olive oil
    Freshly ground black pepper, to taste
    Sweet red pepper slivers and lime wedges, for garnish

Preheat the oven to 350°F.

If necessary, trim dark parts from tuna.

In a small bowl, combine thyme, oil and black pepper into a smooth paste and rub into each piece of fish.

Place fish in a Pyrex baking dish and bake uncovered until cooked through, 30 to 45 minutes, depending on thickness and how you like it cooked.

Place fish on serving platter and serve hot, strewn with pepper slivers, with lime wedges on the side.

Yield: 4 servings

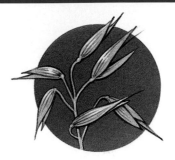

Oatmeal beats other fibers in lowering cholesterol. Its fiber surrounds cholesterol molecules and carts them away.

OAT BRAN MUESLI

½   cup oat bran
1   cup rolled oats
1   cup plain low-fat yogurt
¼   cup unsalted pumpkin seeds
3   bananas, kiwis, apples or oranges, sliced, or a handful of berries

In a medium-size bowl, stir together oat bran, oats and yogurt. (If the mixture is too stiff, add a bit of skim milk to thin it.)

Place mixture in a container, cover and refrigerate overnight.

To serve, place mixture in individual bowls and mix in the seeds or sprinkle them on top, along with fruit.

Yield: 2 servings

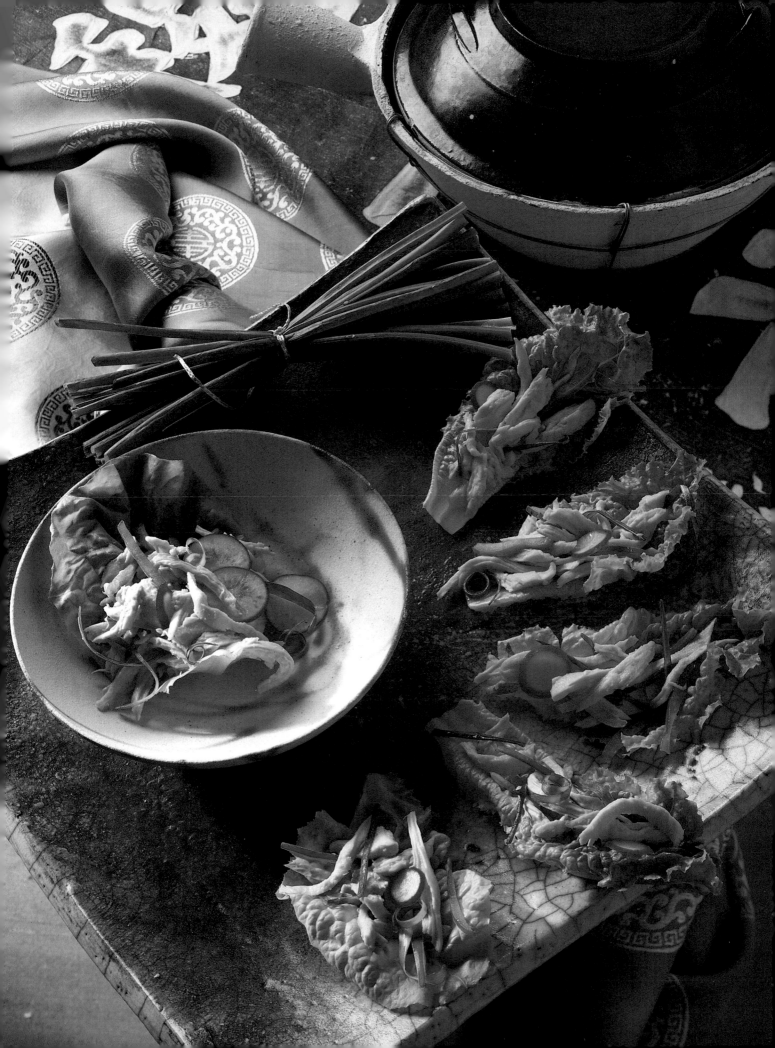

CONSTIPATION

Grunt.

Grunt again, shift your weight.

Groan, arch your back and strain. Feel the blood punch its way up your carotid, the heat building up in your face. Grunt again, and then give up.

Constipation is no fun at all. But this common and uncomfortable condition is more than just bad-joke material for second-rate comedians. It afflicts very large numbers of us for one thing—23 percent of all women and 9 percent of all men, according to researchers from the National Institute of Diabetes and Digestive and Kidney Diseases in Bethesda, Maryland. And even worse, constipation that's left untreated for long periods of time can eventually lead to serious health problems such as diverticulitis—a potentially life-threatening intestinal condition. One theory even implicates it in colon cancer.

The big questions: Are you constipated? And if you are, what can you do about it?

"People have a misconception about constipation," says Brian L. G. Morgan, Ph.D., acting director of the Institute for Human Nutrition at the Columbia University College of Physicians and Surgeons in New York.

"Simply because you haven't gone to the bathroom for two or three days doesn't mean you're constipated. People have different internal clocks regulating these things. But if you have difficulty passing a stool, have to strain to do it or experience discomfort and pain—you're probably constipated."

ARE THERE CONSTIPATING FOODS?

Well—yes and no. Some people find that tea (drunk in large quantities) is a potential problem. But one trouble-maker surfaces more often than others: calcium supplements.

The problem with calcium is that it's not very soluble. The way to avoid problems is either to cut back on your intake, if you're supplementing or eating calcium-rich antacids, or switch to calcium carbonate, which has magnesium salts in it that act as mild laxatives.

Iron supplements commonly prescribed to treat anemia can cause similar problems. One recommended solution is to take them with meals or to lower the dosage.

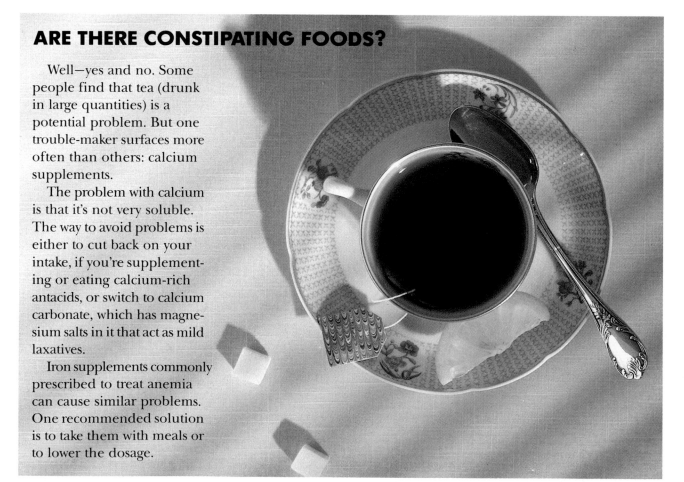

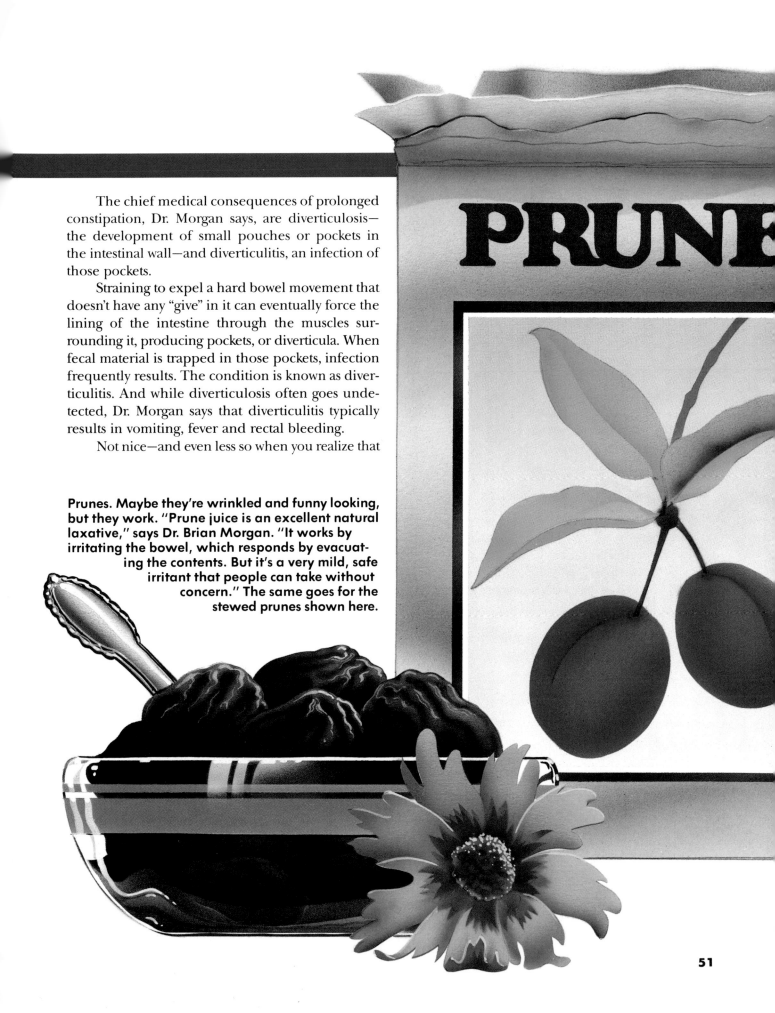

The chief medical consequences of prolonged constipation, Dr. Morgan says, are diverticulosis—the development of small pouches or pockets in the intestinal wall—and diverticulitis, an infection of those pockets.

Straining to expel a hard bowel movement that doesn't have any "give" in it can eventually force the lining of the intestine through the muscles surrounding it, producing pockets, or diverticula. When fecal material is trapped in those pockets, infection frequently results. The condition is known as diverticulitis. And while diverticulosis often goes undetected, Dr. Morgan says that diverticulitis typically results in vomiting, fever and rectal bleeding.

Not nice—and even less so when you realize that

Prunes. Maybe they're wrinkled and funny looking, but they work. "Prune juice is an excellent natural laxative," says Dr. Brian Morgan. "It works by irritating the bowel, which responds by evacuating the contents. But it's a very mild, safe irritant that people can take without concern." The same goes for the stewed prunes shown here.

PRUNE

one-third of all Americans over 45 and two-thirds of those over 60 already have diverticulosis.

But don't panic. There's a lot you can do to prevent the condition or keep it from getting worse. And chances are you'll enjoy doing so, since it mostly involves one of America's favorite pastimes: eating.

THE ROAD TO REGULARITY

Constipation has a variety of causes. Prevention or treatment depends in part on the source of the trouble. Older people, for example, often experience it as a result of a condition known as lazy bowel—intestines that simply don't have the muscle tone to work as hard as they used to. And pregnant women regularly experience constipation when the developing child presses against the intestines.

But for most of us, the villain is distinctly less formidable than age or biology. It's what we eat—or rather, what we don't eat.

"It can be caused by lots of things, but not eating enough fiber or drinking enough liquid are the chief causes," Dr. Morgan says.

Liquid? Right—liquid.

"The thing about fiber and liquid is that it's an absolute waste of time to eat a lot of fiber if you're not getting enough liquid at the same time," Dr. Morgan says. "You eat fiber to add bulk to your stool, but fiber by itself doesn't add much bulk. It becomes bulky by absorbing water. But if you don't drink enough, it *doesn't* bulk up."

Dr. Morgan's basic prescription (drawn from his book, *The Nutrition Prescription*) for treating constipation is simple—add fiber to your diet, enough to bring your daily total to between 20 and 30 grams a day (the amount in a bowl of high-fiber cereal, a serving of broad beans, a baked potato with skin and a pear), and drink at least 1 to 2 quarts of fluid every day. Make that fluid fruit juice, a citrus-ade or just plain old water. Do not rely on coffee, tea or soda to make up your two-quart quota.

Bran and other cereal fibers are the best depluggers, Dr. Morgan says. Fruits and vegetables help to a lesser extent.

One nonfood response to constipation might take a bit more commitment, but Dr. Morgan says it's sometimes as effective as fiber.

"Exercise that uses the upper body is effective in strengthening the intestinal musculature. If you make it a regular part of your life, you'll benefit your interior almost as much as your exterior."

There you have it: cereal, water and sweat. Make the trio part of your health program, and you, too, can start calling yourself "just a regular guy—or gal."

A NATURAL LAXATIVE

For many reasons—the potential for dependency, the principle of the thing—you're not interested in taking one of the many chemical laxatives available today. But you want relief—quickly. What can you do?

Take a natural alternative like Metamucil, says Brian L. G. Morgan, Ph.D., acting director of the Institute for Human Nutrition at the Columbia University College of Physicians and Surgeons in New York.

Made from psyllium seeds, Metamucil is a powdery substance high in water-soluble fiber. You shake the powder into a glass of water or juice and drink it quickly, before it bulks up in the glass. Dr. Morgan says that Metamucil triggers peristalsis—the wavelike contractions that move waste—mechanically, by adding enough bulk to the stool that it presses against the intestinal wall. Recent research, however, has documented a second—and surprising—effect. Metamucil, it seems, also lowers cholesterol levels significantly.

CONSTIPATION
A DAY OF INTENSIVE HEALING

A.M.	**NOON**	**P.M.**

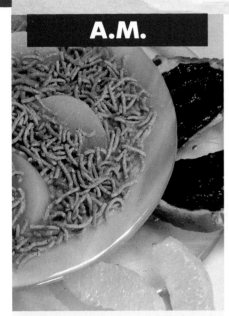 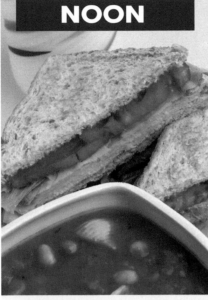 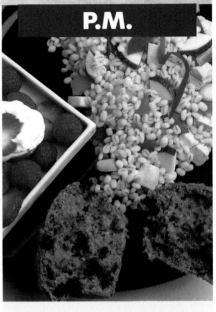

A.M.

Orange
High-fiber bran cereal with
   peaches
Skim milk
Raisin bread with prune
   butter

NOON

Minestrone soup
   (tomato, beans and
   vegetables)
Sliced turkey, romaine
   lettuce and tomato on
   whole wheat bread
Steamed broccoli
Skim milk

P.M.

Barley salad (cold
   cooked barley, peppers,
   zucchini, green onions
   and chicken cubes)
Steamed sweet potatoes,
   pears and raisins
Wheat bran cranberry
   muffin
Strawberries and rasp-
   berries with yogurt
   topping

DISASTER PLATE

Grilled cheeseburger with
   ketchup on white roll
Macaroni, tuna and egg
   salad (white noodles and
   mayonnaise)
Orange soda

   Suppose that for some
reason—you're going

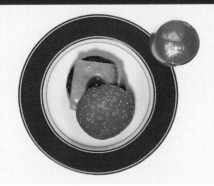

way-y-y-y out there in your
kayak—you want to make
sure you won't have to go to
the bathroom in the near
future. Well, the almost-zero-
fiber, low-fluid meal outlined
here will go a long way
toward plugging you up.

CYSTITIS

Question: What sends American women to the doctor's office most often?

Answer: An uncontrollable, burning urge to go to the bathroom.

That's the main characteristic of cystitis, a bladder or urinary tract infection that forces almost nine million women to seek treatment each year. Men get urinary tract infections, too, but women are struck more often and for different reasons.

Yet there is no reason why even *one* woman should have to visit the doctor for cystitis, says Larrian Gillespie, M.D., clinical instructor in urology at the University of California, Irvine, and author of *You Don't Have to Live with Cystitis.* "Cystitis is something you can easily prevent if armed with common sense and knowledge."

Cystitis is the result of a series of internal events. First, something interferes with the normal functioning of your urinary tract, making it impossible to urinate properly. Because urine does not flow freely, bacteria are trapped in the urinary tract. In that warm, wet, acidic environment, they multiply. The result? A painful bout of cystitis.

Think of urination as a kind of bladder self-cleaning system, as Dr. Gillespie explains in her book. When you go to the bathroom, you naturally flush away *Escherichia coli* (or *E. coli*), the bacteria that usually live in the bowel but can migrate to your urethra. If, however, something prevents the bladder from emptying correctly, the self-cleaning system shuts down.

What is the cause of this mysterious "something" that interferes with normal urinary tract function? A variety of things—a poorly fitted diaphragm or too bulky a tampon, for example. Or the thrusting of your partner's penis during sexual intercourse may cause trauma to your urethra. It could be, too, that your problem is a result of a misaligned lower back or disk pressing on your bladder.

Finally, certain foods can make you sizzle with cystitis pain. Citrus fruits, spicy foods, coffee and alcohol, for example, can all raise the acid level and may stimulate the production of bacterial growth factors, intensifying a burning feeling in the bladder.

When your bladder's on fire, some doctors suggest you reach for that age-old folk remedy— cranberry juice.

Up until recently, it was believed the juice's acid content inhibited bacterial growth. But, says Dr. Gillespie, "Drinking cranberry juice to acidify your urine makes about as much sense as putting out a fire with gasoline." That's because bacteria use a component of acidic urine, called urea, to help them multiply and thrive.

THE ANTICYSTITIS DIET

If you're trying to avoid the burn of cystitis, it's what you *don't* eat that really counts. In addition to the foods already mentioned, Dr. Gillespie says you should try to cut the following acid foods from your diet: apples, apple juice, cantaloupe, carbonated drinks, chilies, grapes, peaches, pineapples, plums, strawberries, tea, tomatoes and vinegar.

Watch out, too, for avocados, bananas, cheese, chocolate, corned beef, lima beans, mayonnaise, aspartame, nuts, onions, prunes, rye bread, saccharin, sour cream, soy sauce and yogurt. These foods are high in tyrosine, tyramine, tryptophan and aspartate —four amino acids that can be irritants.

If you follow these guidelines, which were compiled and published by the Interstitial Cystitis Foundation in Beverly Hills, you may notice results in as little as 24 hours.

What *can* you eat if you've been bothered by cystitis? Well, Dr. Gillespie has some substitution tips. Although raw onions are out, cooked onions in small quantities are fine. Alcohol and wines may be used for flavoring during cooking. Small amounts of the "forbidden fruits" (½ cup of strawberries, for example) should cause you no problems. White chocolate or carob can be substituted for chocolate in any recipe. Processed cheeses that have not been aged—American, ricotta, cottage cheese or cream cheese—can stay on your shopping list, as can fructose, a natural sweetener, and coffee that has had the acid removed.

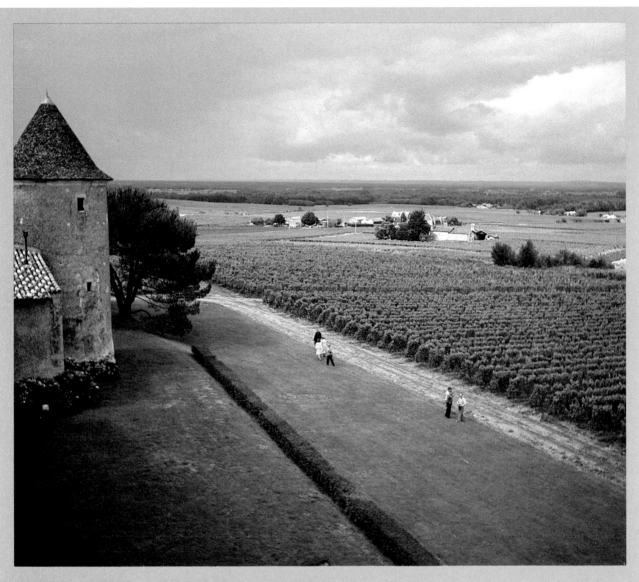

WINES THAT ARE FINE FOR CYSTITIS

When it comes to clinking your glass in a toast, first fill it with the right wine. The choice is not between white and red, but rather between high and low acid. Most French sauternes and late harvest Johannisberg Rieslings are low in acid, as are late harvest dessert wines. In addition, many wines are high in an amino acid called tyramine—also found in cheese, yogurt and beer—that should be avoided by cystitis sufferers. Here is a list of vintages, adapted from *You Don't Have to Live with Cystitis* by Larrian Gillespie, M.D., which are good choices for those wishing to avoid the burn of cystitis.

California Wines

Chateau St. Jean Special Select Late Harvest
Johannisberg Riesling, 1982
Hop Kiln Winery Late Select Botrytis-Shriveled
Berries Weihnachten
Johannisberg Riesling, 1981
Joseph Phelps Vineyards Special Select Late
Harvest Schreurebe

French Wines

Barton and Guestier Sauternes, 1981
Chateau Bastor-Lamontagne Sauternes, 1981
Chateau Nairac Barsac Sauternes, 1980
Chateau Luduraut Sauternes, 1976

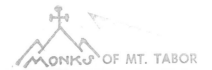

DENTAL PROBLEMS

If the Tooth Fairy gave a dinner party, what would be on the menu?

Phrased a little differently, that question continues to engage the attention of researchers around the world. Archaeological evidence shows that dental cavities were fairly uncommon in antiquity, indicating that rampant tooth decay is somehow a by-product of "civilization." Now scientists are finding how what goes on the modern table can undermine the condition of the modern mouth.

Does *your* smile reflect your daily diet?

You can be certain that it does. Not only does what you eat make a difference, but so do your food combinations and how often you eat.

HOW SWEET IT ISN'T

You've probably heard that dental enemy number one is sugar. Yep, that's the culprit, all right.

When you ingest sugar, you are also providing nourishment for a horde of bacteria that inhabit your mouth and form plaque on your teeth, explains James H. Shaw, Ph.D., professor of nutrition at Harvard School of Dental Medicine.

Within this flourishing bacterial ecosystem live the *Streptococcus mutans,* one of the primary strains of bacteria suspected of causing tooth decay. They thrive on sugar and, as they metabolize it, they create acid, which eats away at your teeth.

PUT THE BITE ON TOOTH DECAY

A number of factors determine whether or not a food can cause cavities: its sugar content, its physical properties and how often it is eaten.

Sugary foods are not limited to the obvious, like candy bars and pastries. Raisins and other dried fruits can be particularly troublesome because they are not only high in sugar but they also stick to your teeth. Eating raisins with other foods such as oatmeal or in a carrot and raisin salad reduces their cavity-causing potential.

Frequent snacking can promote tooth decay by constantly feeding the bacteria that cause the problem. That's why it's important to eat sticky, sugary foods only as part of a regular meal.

NIBBLE AWAY THAT TOOTH DECAY

Say, "Cheese." No, we aren't going to take your picture, but we are going to make your smile pretty.

It seems that cheese is a feast for your teeth. Mark Jensen, D.D.S., Ph.D., of the University of Iowa College of Dentistry, says that what you eat helps control whether or not you will suffer from dental caries. Current research, he says, shows that by encouraging acidity, some snack foods encourage the destructive activities of the caries-causing bacteria that thrive in your mouth. There are also foods, such as cheese, that shut down the bacterial acid factories, neutralizing the conditions that lead to tooth decay.

Dr. Jensen has put together a snack food list that will help you nibble away at tooth decay.

The lists are based on studies done in Sweden and at the Dows Institute for Dental Research in Iowa.

Snack foods on the "Seldom" list should be consumed only with meals. They should be avoided as between-meal snacks. Those on the "Sometimes" list are still problem foods, but not quite as destructive to your teeth.

Seldom: Dates, dried apples, dried apricots, dried pears, cookies, crackers, milk chocolate and potato chips.

Sometimes: Apples, grapes, peaches, pears, apple cider, orange juice and soft drinks.

Go for it: Broccoli, carrots, cauliflower, celery, dill pickles, green peppers, most cheeses, popcorn, almonds, filberts, peanuts, pecans and walnuts.

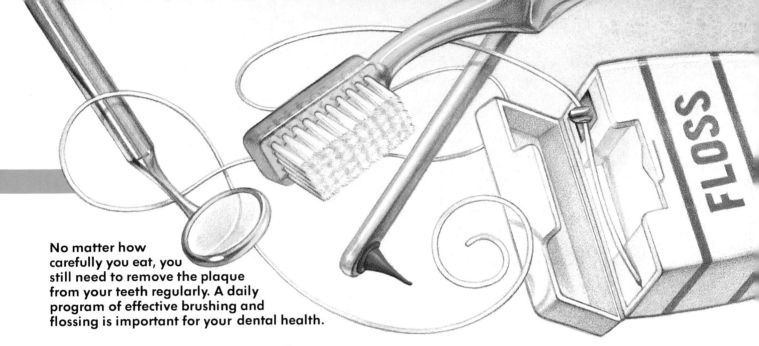

No matter how carefully you eat, you still need to remove the plaque from your teeth regularly. A daily program of effective brushing and flossing is important for your dental health.

WHAT ABOUT GUM DISEASE?

For most adults, the biggest problem isn't cavities, it's periodontal disease—a bacterial infection that attacks gum and eventually bone, loosening teeth.

"The causes of periodontal disease are complicated, and researching it can be frustrating," says Dr. Shaw. And "precious little" research has been done on possible dietary connections.

The kind of plaque that causes periodontal disease is not the same kind of plaque that causes tooth decay. The plaque associated with periodontitis (a form of periodontal disease) lives at or below the gum line.

A somewhat different form of plaque that lives at or above the gum line, however, is responsible for gingivitis. Some believe that this gum inflammation opens the way for periodontitis, says Lawrence Wolinsky, D.M.D., Ph.D., associate professor of oral biology at UCLA's School of Dentistry. So by keeping plaque on your teeth under control, you may help prevent periodontal disease from getting a toehold.

Both Dr. Shaw and Dr. Wolinsky point out that periodontal disease is an infection and that eating a well-balanced diet helps the immune system fight infection. Some experts also recommend making sure that you get enough vitamin C, which helps in the production of collagen in gum tissue.

DIET SODA DILEMMA

Sometimes you think you are doing everything right, but your best intentions can cause you trouble.

Mark Friedman, D.D.S., clinical associate professor of restorative dentistry at the University of Southern California, says a number of dentists are treating people whose tooth enamel has been eroded away.

Based on observation and discussion with other dentists, he now believes that the problem may sometimes be caused by diet soda.

Many soft drinks contain phosphoric and citric acids. These agents can harm tooth enamel but usually don't pose a problem, says Dr. Friedman. What happens with diet drinks is that many people use them as crutches to control their appetites. They'll keep a diet soda on the desk and take a sip every 15 minutes all day long.

If you are one of those people addicted to the diet soda can, Dr. Friedman has some advice: Use a straw. It prevents soda from washing over the teeth and gums.

CHEWING GUM: A STICKY ISSUE

Take this test. Chewing gum (a) causes tooth decay, (b) has no effect on tooth decay, (c) may actually help prevent tooth decay.

Any one of those answers could be correct. When it comes to gum, whether or not it causes dental caries depends on what kind of sweetener it has in it.

Chewing gum sweetened with sugar subjects your teeth to prolonged contact with a caries-causing substance. But current research shows that gum sweetened with sorbitol has little or no ability to cause caries.

And from a study conducted in Finland comes the surprising news that gum sweetened with xylitol may actually provide some protection against dental caries.

DIABETES

The other guy. That's who it happens to. The friendly checker in the supermarket, Alice, is the one who has the stroke. Lou, next door, keels over while shoveling the walk. These kinds of things never happen to *you*.

But this time, it has. There was no one else in your doctor's office when he explained your diagnosis. This time, disease knocked and you answered. You're the one with diabetes mellitus. It's not next door anymore.

Chances are, though, it's on your block. More than ten million people in the United States suffer from non-insulin-dependent diabetes. Robert Silverman, M.D., Ph.D., chief of the Diabetes Programs Branch at the National Institutes of Health, says Type II diabetes usually calls on people with certain similarities.

"Your chances of getting it increase with age—older people get it the most. It's also closely associated with obesity—70 to 90 percent of the people with Type II diabetes are overweight. Also, it seems to be genetically related. So if someone in your family has it, your chances of getting it are higher."

DIABETES DESCRIBED

Adult-onset diabetes, what's called diabetes Type II or non-insulin-dependent diabetes, is not juvenile diabetes grown up. There are differences between the two diseases. Important ones.

"Diabetes is a chronic condition in which the body cannot assimilate its fuel. Diabetes is the body's inability to manage the level of glucose, which is also called blood sugar," explains Dr. Silverman. "The most important regulator of blood sugar is insulin. Insulin is a hormone that removes sugar from the bloodstream and either stores it or makes it available for the body's cells to utilize it. When insulin levels drop, the sugar doesn't make its way into the cells."

Now comes the important difference between the two types of diabetes. "In insulin-dependent diabetes, what we used to call juvenile diabetes, or Type I, the person's pancreas *does not* produce insulin.

"In Type II diabetes, what we used to call adult-onset diabetes, the person's pancreas *does* produce insulin—maybe not in normal amounts, but the insulin is there nonetheless. The problem is, for some reason the body becomes oblivious to the fact that the insulin is present. The person's cells do not respond to it. They literally become insulin resistant."

Diabetes Type II is a "double defeat," according to Aaron Vinik, M.D., professor of internal medicine and surgery at the University of Michigan and chairman of the Nutrition Task Force of the American Diabetes Association. "The person fails to produce insulin in sufficient amounts, and the insulin that is produced is ineffective." But there is hope, he adds. Meal planning combined with a regular exercise program can help the condition. In fact, research has shown that meal planning is crucial.

MANAGING DIABETES WITH DIET

"There's no such thing as a cure for diabetes, but you can control it," says Dr. Vinik. "Of the 10 million or so people in the United States with non-insulin-dependent diabetes, 8.5 million could manage their condition with attention to meal planning."

Hit the pause button here for a second. While many doctors do recommend certain diets, before you decide to try one, please consult with your own physician. Have him design a diet that's especially right for *you*. Dietary changes are not something you should blindly experiment with. (Take the button off pause now.)

Dr. Vinik and the American Diabetes Association recommend "a diet rich in carbohydrates, a high proportion of which are unrefined.

"If you look at the incidence and morbidity from diabetes during World War II rationing, and if you look at countries that normally eat diets of this type, you will find that the incidence of diabetes, and complications from diabetes, decrease. I think people with Type II diabetes will be able to control it with this type of diet," says Dr. Vinik.

He adds that this type of diet is very similar to that now being recommended by the American

Heart Association—low in fat (especially saturated fat) and high in carbohydrates. "This diet shouldn't be regarded as a diet exclusively for diabetics, but as a healthier way of eating for the whole population."

The American Diabetes Association has just come out with new nutritional recommendations for people with diabetes Type II. Dr. Vinik says that there are "major differences" between these new recommendations and those published in the past. "Now we recommend that 55 to 60 percent of your total dietary intake come from carbohydrates. We also suggest that you get upwards of 40 grams of fiber daily." (This is the amount in a cup each of brown rice, baked beans and blackberries, as well as a bran muffin, five prunes and a serving of spinach.)

"People also need to reduce their total intake of fats to not more than 30 percent of total calories, keeping cholesterol levels low. We also recommend that people reduce their salt intake and alcohol consumption and exercise regularly. A diet like this appears to protect the pancreas so it can make more insulin. In addition, it seems to increase the effectiveness of the insulin."

What's good for your pancreas may be vitally important for other organs as well.

CONTROLLING DIABETES COMPLICATIONS

People don't die from diabetes—but they can die from complications brought on by the disease. Dr. Vinik believes a diet like the one recommended will help control those complications. "For people with Type II diabetes, there's at least a fivefold increase in the risk of vascular problems such as heart disease, stroke or gangrene. Evidence is showing that this type of diet is orientated to diminishing those complications."

Marian Eschleman is the director of nutrition at the Princeton Diabetes Treatment and Education Center, which is located in Princeton, New Jersey. She counsels patients about their dietary habits, and she says she tries to tailor the diet to fit their individual lifestyles.

READ

Please. If you have diabetes, changing your diet is *not* something that should be taken lightly.

"If you have diabetes Type II and you're on insulin or taking an oral hypoglycemic, you should definitely see your physician before you change your diet," says Robert Silverman, M.D., Ph.D.

"The dosage you're taking now has been calculated according to the amount of food you are now eating. Changing your diet without changing the dosage could drop your blood-sugar levels too low, causing you to pass out, or worse," he warns.

Dr. Silverman also recommends that you make it a practice to see your physician not just for specific changes but also as an ongoing partnership in managing your diabetes.

"Eat more dried beans, peas and lentils," she tells her patients. "Add more whole grain bread, cereal and crackers to your diet. Also, eat more fruits and vegetables."

Eschleman gives them another dietary tip: "Instead of skipping breakfast or loading up at dinner, we try to get them to distribute the food they eat more evenly over the day. People are very weight-conscious before 5 o'clock, but after that they throw caution to the wind. They eat large dinners and continue eating till they go to bed. We try to get them to spread their eating out over the day."

The weight-consciousness is crucial. If you're looking for the bottom line in helping to control your diabetes, you should start looking at your waistline. Dr. Silverman says that losing weight is the key to controlling Type II diabetes.

"When a diabetic person who is obese loses weight, very often their diabetes markedly improves. The object of dietary therapy of diabetes mellitus [Type II] is primarily to get the person to lose weight. Based on the data available, the evidence clearly shows that controlling your weight is crucial," he says.

FOOD EXCHANGES FOR A VARIED DIET

In diabetes, there is no such thing as "one diet fits all." However, the American Diabetes Association has developed a *basic* menu of healthy food choices that you can use to help plan your meals. They recommend that each day you should have at least four choices from the starch/bread group, five meat or meat substitute choices, two vegetable choices, two fruit choices, two skim milk choices and not more than three fat choices. The meal plan adds up to about 1,200 calories a day. In addition, they recommend that you eat smaller servings of meat—choosing fish, poultry and lean red meat over other selections. Prepare all meats by roasting, baking or broiling. Trim off all fat and remove skin from poultry. Be careful, too, of added sauces or gravy.

Also avoid all other sources of fat. Avoid fried foods, and don't add fat during cooking. Eat fewer high-fat foods such as cold cuts, bacon, sausage, hot dogs, butter, margarine, nuts, salad dressings, lard and solid shortening.

In addition to cutting fat, increase the amount of high-fiber foods you eat, such as legumes, whole grains, vegetables and fruits.

At the same time, they recommend that you watch the amount of salt and sugar that you eat. Don't keep a saltshaker on the table, reduce the amount of salt you add while cooking, and avoid foods that taste salty. Also eat fewer high-salt foods like canned soup, ham, sauerkraut, hot dogs and pickles. Avoid regular soft drinks, table sugar, honey, syrup, jam, jelly, candy, sweet rolls, fruit canned in syrup, gelatin desserts, cake with icing, pie or other sweets. Instead, choose fresh fruit (or fruit canned in its own juice or water) and use noncaloric sweeteners instead of sugar.

If you use this plan as a basis and work with your physician, you should be able to custom-tailor a diet for your own needs.

VEGETABLES

Each of these equals one vegetable choice (25 calories).
½ cup cooked vegetables
1 cup raw vegetables
½ cup tomato/vegetable juice

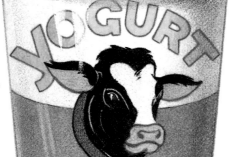

MILK

Each of these equals one milk choice. The calories vary for each choice.
1 cup skim milk (90 calories)
1 cup low-fat milk (120 calories)
8-ounce carton plain low-fat
  yogurt (120 calories)

FATS

Each of these equals one fat choice (45 calories).
1 teaspoon margarine, oil
  or mayonnaise
2 teaspoons diet margarine or
  diet mayonnaise
1 tablespoon salad dressing
2 tablespoons reduced-calorie
  salad dressing

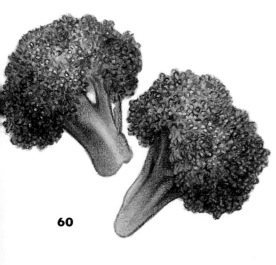

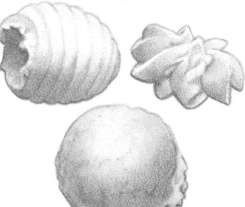

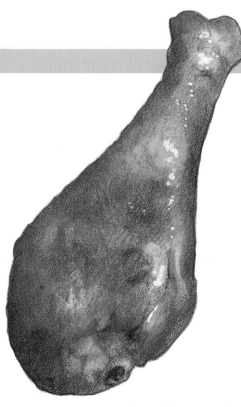

MEAT AND SUBSTITUTES

Each of these equals one meat choice (75 calories).

1 ounce cooked poultry, fish or meat
¼ cup cottage cheese
¼ cup salmon or tuna, water-packed
1 tablespoon peanut butter
1 egg (limit to 3 per week)
1 ounce low-fat cheese, such as mozzarella or ricotta

Each of these equals two meat choices (150 calories).

1 small chicken leg or thigh
½ cup cottage cheese or tuna, water-packed

Each of these equals three meat choices (225 calories).

1 small pork chop
1 small hamburger
cooked meat, about the size of a deck of cards
½ of a whole chicken breast
1 medium fish fillet

STARCHES

Each of these equals one starch choice (80 calories).

½ cup pasta or barley
⅓ cup rice or cooked dried beans and peas
1 small potato (or ½ cup mashed)
½ cup starchy vegetables (corn, peas or winter squash)
1 slice bread or 1 roll
½ English muffin, bagel or hamburger/hot dog bun
½ cup cooked cereal
¾ cup dry cereal, unsweetened
4–6 crackers
3 cups popcorn, unbuttered, not cooked in oil

FRUITS

Each of these equals one fruit choice (60 calories).

1 medium fresh fruit
1 cup berries or melon
½ cup canned fruit in juice or without sugar
½ cup fruit juice
¼ cup dried fruit

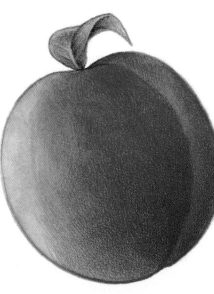

EXTRAS

Free foods (less than 20 calories per serving).

Bouillon without fat*
Ketchup (1 tablespoon)
Coffee/tea
Diet, calorie-free drinks
Diet syrup
Hot sauces
Lemon
Lime
Low-sugar jam/jelly (2 teaspoons)
Mustard
Nonstick pan sprays
Raw vegetables
    cabbage, celery, cucumbers, green beans, green onions, mushrooms, radishes and zucchini
Salad greens
    lettuce, romaine and spinach
Soy sauce*
Spices/herbs
Sugar-free gum
Sugar substitutes
Unsweetened gelatin
Unsweetened pickles*
Vinegar
Wine (¼ cup used in cooking)
Worcestershire sauce

*High in salt.

DIET AND WORLD HEALTH

GREENLAND

The Eskimos of Greenland eat almost a pound of fish a day, and research suggests that's why they have been shown to have significantly lower levels of cholesterol, triglycerides, and fatal heart disease than Westerners.

ALASKA AND NORTHERN CANADA

The Eskimos in this part of the Far North have unprecedented levels of tooth decay. They also eat more sugar than almost any other population in the world. Once, when they lived almost solely on meat and fish, tooth decay was nearly unknown.

ITALY AND GREECE

Lately, a lot of us have added a new oil to our diet—olive oil—in order to cut levels of serum cholesterol. Well, Mediterranean people have used olive oil for centuries. And a 15-year, seven-country study links their diet with lower heart disease death rates.

TOGO

When researchers screened 1,381 natives of the West African villages of Kati and Agbave, they didn't find a single case of diabetes. The villagers' diet, high in complex carbohydrates and fiber, (an amazing 84 percent of total calories were from carbs, mainly in the form of root vegetables and corn) may account for the disease's rarity.

BRAZIL

Perhaps you're not quite up to catching your own fish as the Brazilian tribe of Upper Xingu Indians do. But a low-sodium diet like theirs, including plenty of fresh fish, vegetables and fruits, may, in fact, help to keep blood pressure low. Heart disease, ulcers, hernias, appendicitis and diverticular disease are also rare among the Xingu.

INTRODUCTION

If the U.S. government had an *Ate* Department instead of a *State* Department, a globe-hopping diplomat might send a top-secret cable like this one:

GARLIC PREVENTS STOMACH CANCER IN CHINA STOP DIABETES LOWER AMONG YAM-EATING ABORIGINES STOP KENYANS DON'T GET HEMORRHOIDS STOP CHANGING MY DIET TODAY STOP

Lucky for you, though, this kind of information isn't classified: Take a world tour with the food scientists who've investigated states of good health.

CHINA

Two counties in China's Shardong province are alike in every feature but one: Quixia has a death rate from stomach cancer ten times higher than that of Gangshan. Why the difference? People in Gangshan eat large quantities of garlic, which may reduce the formation of cancer-causing substances in the stomach.

JAPAN

When Japanese migrate to the United States, their low incidences of breast, colon and lung cancers don't usually make it past customs. A change in diet, say researchers, is the reason. When they swap their low-milk, little-meat, high-fish, low-fat diet for a Western one, cancer rates shoot up.

PAPUA, NEW GUINEA

The next time your doctor tells you to cut down on salt and fat, think of the people of Murapin. They've followed that advice for hundreds of years, and they have virtually no coronary heart disease.

UGANDA, KENYA AND TANZANIA

In one respect, residents of sub-Sahara Africa are luckier than one in two Americans over age 50—they rarely seem to suffer from the itch and pain of hemorrhoids. One speculation as to why focuses on their high-fiber diet.

And for those of you who live with high blood pressure, perhaps a sweet potato or two would be in order. The reason: high potassium, which may be part of the explanation why primitive communities in Uganda, Kenya and Tanzania have relatively little hypertension.

AUSTRALIA

You might not find foods like wattle seeds or cheeky yams at the supermarket, but these carbohydrates may have protected Australian aborigines from diabetes. A tip for the rest of us: Eat more legumes.

DIVERTICULOSIS

What do monthly car payments, stock market slumps and diverticulosis have in common? They're all unfortunate by-products of Western civilization. Tarzan, after all, swung around the jungle just fine on a vine, with no need for a Ford. Traders in the old days made dependable deals in skins and furs, not risky deals in securities and futures. And not so long ago, Americans made their meals of grains and fresh fruits and vegetables, not the refined and processed foods that today are considered a major contributor to—among other physical ills—diverticulosis.

If you live in Africa, Asia or any country with an "undeveloped" diet, your chances of having diverticular disease are quite low. We Westerners, however, get it frequently, especially as we grow older. Researchers estimate that at least one out of every three Americans over 60 has it.

Diverticular disease usually occurs in the colon, the last lap of intestines that form the winding roads of your digestive tract. What happens is that strange little pouches, called diverticula, form along the colon's inside walls.

HOW THINGS CHANGE

In the past, people with diverticulosis were advised to steer clear of high-fiber foods on the theory that roughage acted like an abrasive, eroding the blood vessels and causing inflammation in the intestinal lining. Today doctors believe fiber's increased bulk relieves strain on the colon's muscle walls.

1950s: Restricted Foods	1980s: Recommended Foods
Bran cereals	Bran cereals
Whole wheat bread	Whole wheat bread
Brown rice	Brown rice
Fresh fruits	Fresh fruits
Raw vegetables	Raw vegetables

The cause of these pouches is still a medical mystery, but the most popular theory is that it has something to do with increased pressure in the intestinal tract, as well as decreased resistance in the bowel wall.

MOTHER NATURE UNDER STRAIN

"It seems to be related to pressure in the intestinal tract," says Samuel Klein, M.D., an assistant professor of gastroenterology at the University of Texas. "When the pressure inside the colon is greater than the tensile strength of the colon wall, outpouches form." The condition occurs more frequently if a person experiences even more increased pressure—such as when someone is constipated. The incidence increases, too, when the strength of the intestinal wall decreases—as it does when we grow older, or if someone has certain diseases of the connective tissue.

Increased pressure? Resistance in the bowel? Sounds painful. Yet you could have diverticulosis at this very moment and not feel a thing. As many as 80 percent of its victims have no symptoms. But don't worry. "If it's not bothering you, there's no reason at all to be concerned with it," says Dr. Klein.

The real problem occurs for the remaining 20 percent of cases, in which the diverticula, or pouches, cause internal bleeding or become inflamed in a very serious, very painful form of the condition called diverticulitis.

If you are one of the more fortunate 80 percent, there really is no treatment for the disease. Dr. Klein suggests that "increasing dietary fiber intake would be reasonable." Other studies suggest that high fiber may even prevent the formation of diverticula in the first place.

HOW HIGH IS "HIGH FIBER"?

"The average American diet contains about 10 to 20 grams of fiber per day. For most people, then, it would be prudent to increase it to 25 to 35 grams," says Dr. Klein. "One additional serving of a cereal, a legume such as beans, a vegetable and a fruit daily

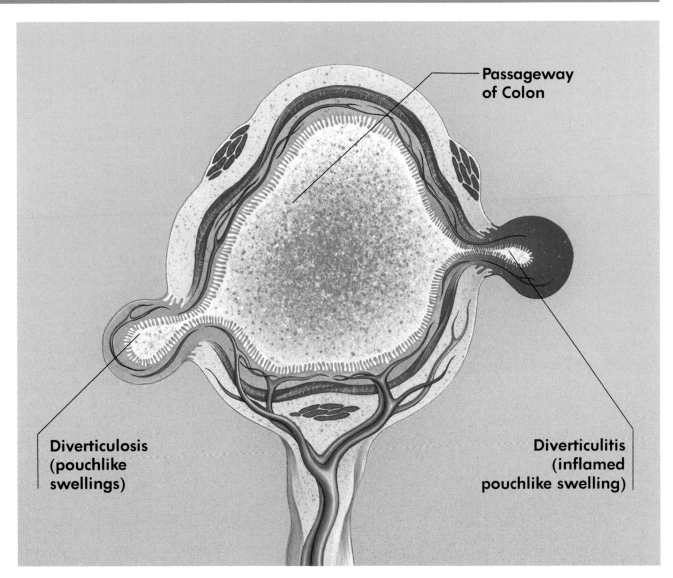

Passageway of Colon

Diverticulosis (pouchlike swellings)

Diverticulitis (inflamed pouchlike swelling)

will increase your fiber intake by about 15 to 20 grams," he says.

Add to that plenty of bran, says Marvin Schuster, M.D., chief of digestive diseases and professor of medicine at Francis Scott Key Medical Center. "Eat more all-bran cereal, whole wheat bread and brown rice. And drink more water to increase bulk."

Look in your grocery store for foods prepared with whole grains, including whole grain flours, crackers, waffles, pastas and even desserts, or try recipes of your own. Also high in fiber are beans in all their varieties, peas, potatoes and vegetable soups.

Bulk up your diet over a period of several weeks. Otherwise, you may find yourself with a disturbing case of bloating, flatulence or diarrhea, says Dr. Klein. He also notes a very important exception to all this high-fiber talk: Absolutely *do not* eat fiber if you're having a diverticulitis attack, when your colon needs a vacation from digestion. Drink lots of water and juice instead. When things get back to normal, head for the high fiber. Who knows? That last attack might really be your last.

ENERGY

ESCAPE FROM THE SUGAR TRAP

Sure, sugar gives you a jolt—but you pay for it later. It doesn't take long before your sugar high becomes a sugar low. Eat nonsugary complex carbohydrates instead to get more staying power.

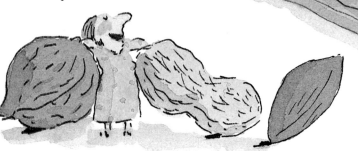

DON'T EAT A BIG MEAL LATE AT NIGHT

You probably won't be able to burn off the calories as quickly by bedtime as you would earlier in the day. Get in the habit of eating most of your calories earlier in the day, or plan on an early supper.

SKIP ALCOHOL AFTER DINNER

Booze, contrary to popular myth, interferes with sound sleep.

GET A BUZZ FROM THE B'S

B vitamins help convert proteins, carbohydrates and fats to fuel. Without them, you're sunk.

GRAB A HANDFUL OF NUTS

If you feel fatigued, especially after exercising, you may have what one medical expert calls the mineral blues—a deficiency of potassium and magnesium in muscle cells. Both minerals can be lost through sweat. When stores drop below normal, even a mild deficiency can bring on fatigue. Both potassium and magnesium are abundant in nuts and soybeans.

TAKE C AND SEE

Several studies suggest that people whose diets are lacking vitamin C grow fatigued more quickly than those whose C intakes are high. Aside from C's immediate effects, there's a bonus: It helps increase your absorption of dietary iron, sometimes as much as 300 percent. Realize that C will energize you only if your lack of energy is the result of a nutrient deficiency.

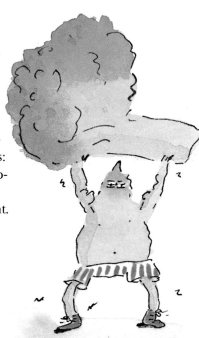

EAT A LIGHT LUNCH

Eating a heavy lunch can make you a victim of postprandial dip, characterized by a drop in body temperature, blood sugar, work efficiency and mood. In many countries lunch is followed by a siesta. If you can't get a daily nap written into your benefit package, eat lightly.

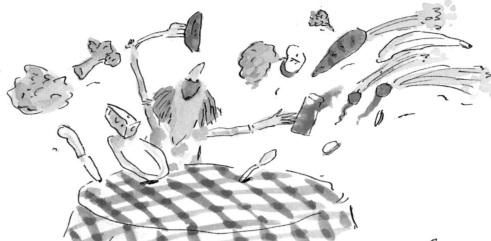

DON'T SKIP MEALS

If you do, you'll only be hungrier later. Then, when you finally do sit down to eat, you'll likely wind up eating more than you should. For a smoother flow of energy, try to spread out those calories more evenly during the course of the day.

EAT A VARIETY OF FOODS

Avoid diet plans that force you to live on one specific kind of food, like grapefruit or pasta. We need a wide variety of nutrients from all kinds of food. And we should vary the mix of specific foods from day to day. No one food supplies you with all the nutrients you need for good health and high energy.

EAT A GOOD BREAKFAST

Depending on how much you toss and turn, you can use up 500 to 600 calories getting a good night's sleep. Even if you don't wake up hungry, your body has still been depleted of the vitamins and minerals that give you the energy to tackle a brand-new day.

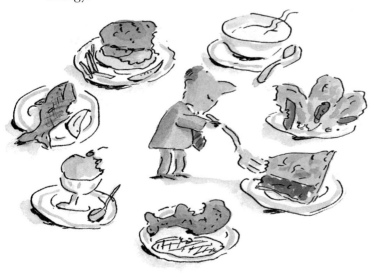

DRINK COFFEE ONLY AT TEATIME

You may think it gives you zip, but coffee triggers an insulin reaction, just as sugar does. After an hour of manic energy, it can leave you with a mild case of low blood sugar. A cup in the morning can interfere with your circadian rhythms, according to Charles Ehret, Ph.D., senior scientist at the Argonne National Laboratory. At different phases of the day, the body's internal alarm clock raises and lowers your blood pressure and body temperature, triggers thousands of chemicals to turn on and off, and makes you feel dexterous or clumsy. A better time to drink coffee, if you must, is English teatime, between 3:30 and 5:00 P.M.

FIBROCYSTIC BREAST DISEASE

Sheila never had to look at a calendar to know when her period was nearing. "My breasts would swell, ache and become lumpy right up until my period started," she says. "Now the painful lumps are always there—I can't even sleep on my stomach anymore!"

Sheila has fibrocystic disease, a catchall term for lumpy breasts, a condition that half of all women experience. Sixty percent, in fact, experience pain that's severe enough to send them to the doctor sometime in their lives.

If that's not bad enough, these tender lumps may also prevent women from practicing routine breast exams. And that, says John Minton, M.D., Ph.D., professor of surgery at Ohio State University College of Medicine, could be disastrous. The reason? A certain number of women with fibrocystic breast disease—those with a personal or family history of cancer—may have lumps that are cancerous. "It's important to eliminate the painful lumps," says Dr. Minton, for health's sake as much as comfort.

THE CAUSE OF BREAST LUMPS

Most normal breast lumps occur just before menstruation, when fluctuating amounts of the female hormones are released. Breasts may swell and form lumps that subside when the period starts.

But sometimes, as in Sheila's case, the painful lumps don't go away. Why? Supposedly, the hormones have become imbalanced. "The breast is hormonally programmed to make or not make milk," explains Dr. Minton. "If it receives mixed messages, the breast cells may produce fluid when there's nowhere for it to go. So it accumulates and causes discomfort. Fluid-filled cysts may form."

Just what makes the hormones go haywire? Dr. Minton has traced part of the problem to consuming coffee, tea, colas or chocolate. These foods contain caffeine and other methylxanthines, substances that produce biochemical signals that activate breast hormones and promote cyst fluid.

According to Dr. Minton's studies, when women with fibrocystic breast disease gave up coffee and cola, they also said good-bye to painful breast lumps.

SHOULD YOU QUIT COFFEE?

Since Dr. Minton's findings, several other studies have failed to find a clear caffeine connection to fibrocystic breast disease. Yet, even without conclusive scientific evidence, many doctors admit that eliminating methylxanthines does seem to work for some women.

"It's a solution that appears to offer relief for breast lumps and certainly involves little risk," reports David Rose, M.D., chief of the Division of Nutrition and Endocrinology at the American Health Foundation.

To see if cutting out caffeine eases your breast lumps, Dr. Minton suggests you completely abstain from coffee (and other products that contain caffeine) for at least two months (or four months if you are over 30). It takes that long to reduce swelling and pain, although the lumps themselves may not subside for two years.

If, after trying these measures, you still have painful lumps, says Dr. Rose, you might want to cut back on fatty foods. Studies conducted by the American Health Foundation found that when women with fibrocystic breast disease reduced their fat consumption by 20 percent, their levels of prolactin went down. Prolactin is one of the hormones that contribute to cysts. The women reported that their breast pain decreased or disappeared.

Here are a few more dietary adjustments that may reduce breast pain:
- Eat fiber-rich foods. Fiber may help escort excess estrogen out of the body so breasts don't become overstimulated.
- Season without salt. Salt promotes fluid retention and breast swelling.
- Try eliminating tyramines. According to Dr. Minton, tyramines, a natural substance found in foods such as cheeses, wines, spices, nuts, mushrooms and bananas can abnormally stimulate breast hormones.

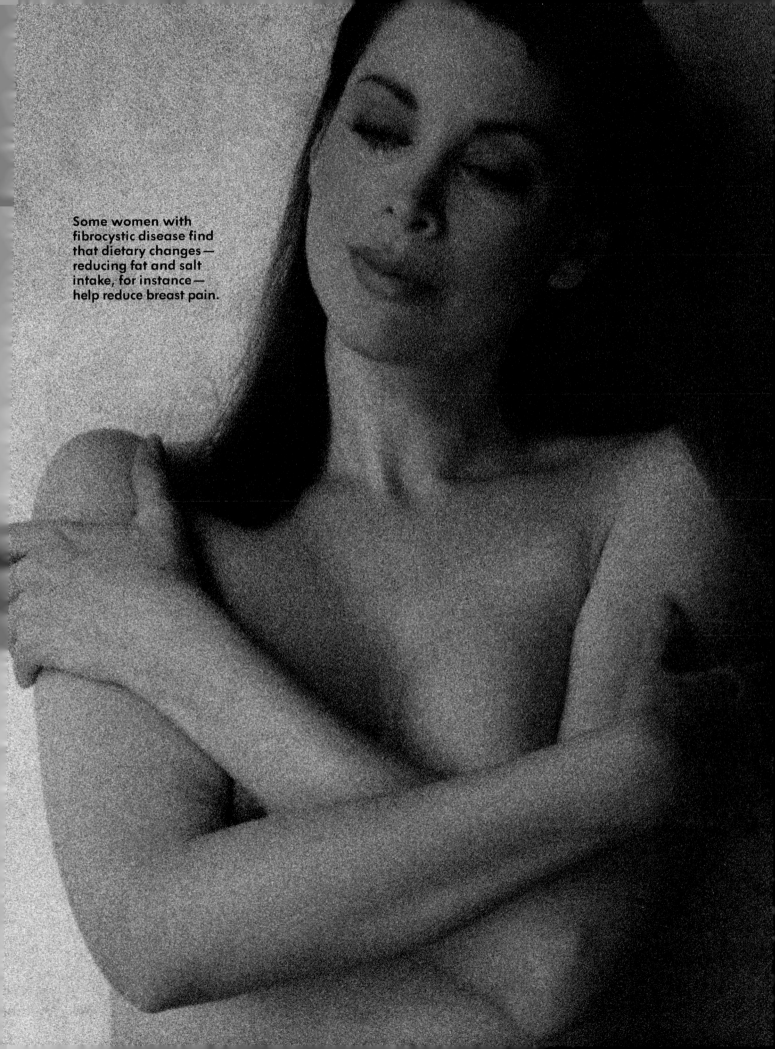

Some women with fibrocystic disease find that dietary changes—reducing fat and salt intake, for instance—help reduce breast pain.

FRINGE DIETS AND BEYOND

You know that if you eat fatty meats, you risk clogging up your arteries, and if you eat green vegetables, you reduce your risk of cancer. But did you know that some people believe there may be a connection between eggplant and arthritis? Between food dyes and kids who act obnoxious? Between honey and your emotional equilibrium?

On this and the following pages, we take a brief but discerning look at five meal plans that each promise a healthier you. We call them fringe because these diets are (with one exception) the nutritional equivalent of religious cults. Some people believe in them passionately. But most people—and that includes most doctors and researchers—would prefer not to eat while bowing down.

You already know that tobacco is bad for you. But are you aware that other members of the nightshade family—eggplant, tomato, potato and most peppers—contain poisons that may give you arthritis or may possibly kill you? That's what horticulturist Dr. Norman Childers says, but few doctors agree.

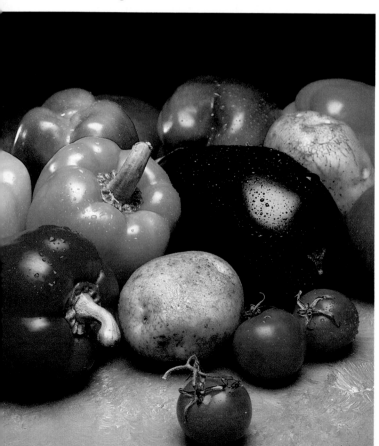

THE NO-NIGHTSHADES DIET

Norman F. Childers, Ph.D., is involved in a family feud. The object of his animosity is a family of plants and trees called the Solanaceae, or, more commonly, the nightshades. According to Dr. Childers, this family commits a crime with millions of victims: arthritis.

If you have arthritis, Dr. Childers claims that by eliminating nightshades, the chances are better than seven in ten that you'll get better. If you don't have arthritis, Dr. Childers says giving up nightshades is the best preventive measure you can take.

What's the matter? You can't remember sinking your fork into a bowl of steaming nightshades lately? Sure you do. You've probably eaten nightshade fried, sliced, diced or tucked into a sandwich several times in the last week alone. You may have smoked some as well.

The nightshade family, you see, includes not only the deadly belladonna but also the tomato and potato, eggplant, all peppers except black pepper, and tobacco. Dr. Childers, a horticulturist who is currently a professor of fruit crops at the University of Florida, says that these nightshades contain small amounts of various toxins that affect the body in numerous and nefarious ways. He cites high blood pressure and cancer, but—above all—aching joints.

His own aches and pains led Dr. Childers to wean himself off nightshades back in the 1960s. He got better, and he wrote a book about it entitled *Arthritis: Childers' Diet to Stop It!* His support in the medical community is nearly nonexistent.

But at least one physician gives Dr. Childers some credit. "Since he came out with his diet, I've suggested it to 60, maybe 70, patients for whom it has worked. There are also some for whom it hasn't," says Jonathan Wright, M.D., of Kent, Washington. "Considering that you only have to give up four vegetables on Childers's diet, it's certainly worth being given a chance," he says.

But giving up a few vegetables may no longer be enough. "We've searched out the main culprit in nightshades and discovered it is vitamin D_3," says Dr. Childers. Naturally found in nightshades, it is now being used in place of vitamin D_2 to fortify milk and some other products. "In high dosages," he says, "vitamin D_3 makes a very effective rat poison."

THE FEINGOLD DIET

Our great-grandparents didn't have to concern themselves with food additives and artificial colorings. Back then, nuts were brown, cherries were red and vanilla ice cream was always white. Life was simple.

Today, we eat kaleidoscopic snack cakes and breakfast cereals, psychedelic candies and gums, grass green cherries, lipstick red pistachios and tutti-frutti ice cream of hues too brilliant to be found in nature.

The government says most of these artificial colorings are safe. But some say they have seen proof of these chemicals' harmful effects. One is Jane Hersey of Alexandria, Virginia. That's why she turned to the Feingold Diet.

Jane Hersey's daughter, Laura, was 6 years old at the time. "She was unpredictable; she'd get terribly upset for no reason; she once dumped a Slurpee over her head and even into her sneakers. I asked myself if there was brain damage, or if she was emotionally disturbed," says Hersey.

"And then," she says, "a neighbor passed along Dr. Feingold's book."

Jane Hersey read *Why Your Child Is Hyperactive,* by Ben Feingold, M.D., a pediatrician specializing in childhood allergies, who turned author in 1975.

She read about colorings, artificial flavorings and preservatives in food and medications. And she read about salicylate, an aspirinlike substance found in most fruits, coffee, tea and a few vegetables. These are responsible not only for hyperactivity in many children but for a broad range of health problems in children as well as adults, Dr. Feingold said.

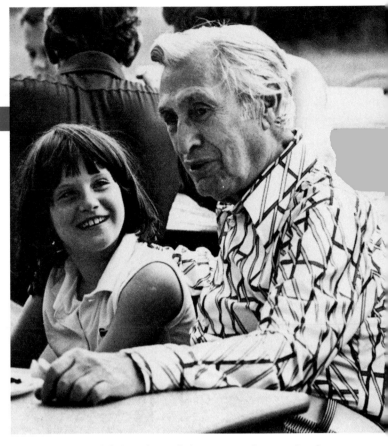

Dr. Ben Feingold developed the somewhat radical theory that modern food additives cause bratty kids.

THE DIET IN ACTION

Jane Hersey tried Dr. Feingold's rather complicated salicylate- and additive-free diet on Laura. Within days, says Hersey, Laura's hyperactivity stopped. Harry Hersey, father and husband, also tried the diet, and the migraine headaches he had suffered for years stopped.

Today the executive director of The Feingold Association of the United States, Jane Hersey says 200,000 families use the diet.

Its popularity with parents and some professionals aside, the medical establishment is skeptical. The official word from the American Academy of Pediatrics is that Dr. Feingold "fails to provide scientific rigor needed for upholding such assertions."

Believers admit there is a lack of scientific proof, but they contend the diet's record speaks for itself. Critics contend that only rarely will the diet make a difference in a child's behavior. More often, they say, the Feingold parents' increased attention to the hyperactive child is what really is at work in curing the hyperactivity.

THE MACROBIOTIC DIET

To the casual observer, the standard macrobiotic diet seems quite simple: whole grain cereals, which make up the lion's share of each meal, supplemented by vegetables or beans or occasionally by fish or fruit. But up close, the macrobiotic diet is anything but simple.

"It's a way of eating incorporated into a way of life," says Richard Donze, D.O., a family practitioner at the Pritikin Longevity Center near Philadelphia. He explains (but does not endorse) the diet, saying that its ultimate achievement is balance. The balance is between the two basic forces of the universe, yin (expansion) and yang (contraction), as well as a balance among the five basic elements—water, earth, wood, fire and metal.

Not everyone can achieve balance by eating the same foods. The diet will change according to a person's age, sex, activity and cultural background, say its followers. The diet also will change as do the seasons and the temperature. If you are a woman, for instance (women are yin, men are yang), you live in a cold climate (cold is yin), and you are doing

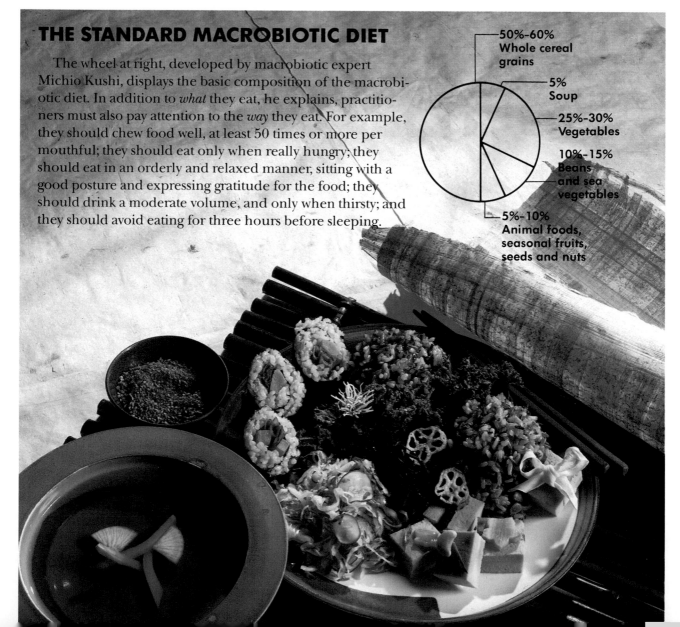

THE STANDARD MACROBIOTIC DIET

The wheel at right, developed by macrobiotic expert Michio Kushi, displays the basic composition of the macrobiotic diet. In addition to *what* they eat, he explains, practitioners must also pay attention to the *way* they eat. For example, they should chew food well, at least 50 times or more per mouthful; they should eat only when really hungry; they should eat in an orderly and relaxed manner, sitting with a good posture and expressing gratitude for the food; they should drink a moderate volume, and only when thirsty; and they should avoid eating for three hours before sleeping.

- 50%–60% Whole cereal grains
- 5% Soup
- 25%–30% Vegetables
- 10%–15% Beans and sea vegetables
- 5%–10% Animal foods, seasonal fruits, seeds and nuts

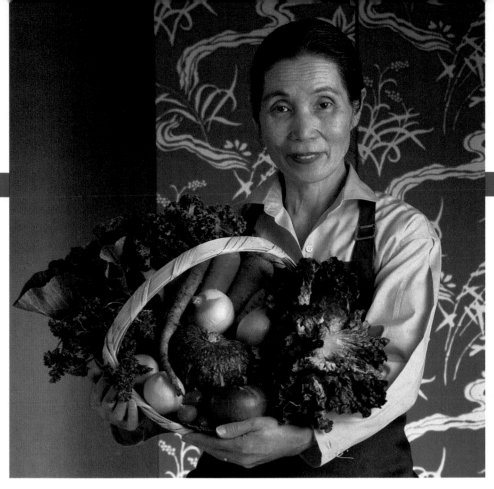

Aveline Kushi, with her husband, Michio Kushi, helped to introduce the macrobiotic diet to Europe and the United States. She also develops macrobiotic recipes that use whole grains and fresh vegetables, such as those shown here.

intellectual work (yin again), in order to achieve balance you would probably do well to eat more fish (yang) and less honey (yin).

Determining which foods are yang and which are yin is somewhat systematic but a bit whimsical as well, says Dr. Donze. One determination is where a particular food is grown (the tropics are yang), what its texture is (yin is soft, yang is hard) and whether it is grown under or above the ground (growing underground makes foods yang).

CURING LEPROSY IN TEN DAYS

If macrobiotics can be compared to a religion, then its most notable prophet was undoubtedly the Japanese-born (now deceased) George S. Ohsawa. In his book *Zen Macrobiotics,* Ohsawa describes the diet's potential: "I have seen thousands of incurable diseases such as asthma, diabetes, epilepsy, leprosy and paralyses of all kinds cured by . . . macrobiotics in ten days or a few weeks," he wrote.

Offering an explanation of these alleged healing qualities, macrobiotic author and teacher Alex Jack of Dallas explains, "The macrobiotic diet is in balance and harmony with nature and the environment around us. As such, it helps strengthen our natural immunity to some of the diseases of modern civilization."

These claims got a lot of national attention in 1978. In that year, a friend and colleague of Dr. Donze, Anthony Sattilaro, M.D., former president of Philadelphia's Methodist Hospital, announced that he had been miraculously cured of his advanced prostate cancer, in part due to a macrobiotic diet. (Dr. Sattilaro has since written a book about it: *Recalled by Life.*)

Macrobiotics also has received some bad publicity, including reports of a number of cases of rickets among children on the diet. Dr. Donze says the parents of these children didn't correctly apply macrobiotic principles, but others question the principles themselves.

"People who are highly trained in nutrition could certainly give themselves a nutritionally sufficient diet, given the macrobiotic emphasis on grains and vegetables," says Rita Storey, a registered dietitian and former professor of nutrition at California State University and an officer of the American Dietetic Association. "But the diet is complicated and difficult for someone with limited knowledge to follow," she adds. Yet, she wouldn't dismiss the Japanese-origin macrobiotic diet as a "bad" diet. "It doesn't make a lot of sense to me, but it comes from an Eastern approach, and that process of thinking isn't quite the same as ours," she says.

THE STONE AGE DIET

Human beings are designed to walk rather than fly, crawl or slither along on their bellies. Are we also designed to digest certain foods better than others? Yes, according to S. Boyd Eaton, M.D., associate professor of radiology at Emory University Medical School. He says that our metabolism is every bit as genetically programmed as are our legs and our spine, and those of us eating typical American diets, he says, are, in effect, slithering.

"We today have a mismatch between our genes and our lifestyle that could account for more than half the deaths in the United States," says Dr. Eaton. The most common diseases of the day, such as heart disease, hypertension, diabetes and some cancers, he says, can be prevented by a return to the more traditional diet of humankind.

In Dr. Eaton's book *The Paleolithic Prescription* (written with anthropologists Marjorie Shostak and Melvin Konner, M.D., Ph.D.), he recommends not woolly mammoth steaks and saber-toothed-tiger burgers, but lots of fresh fruits and vegetables, lean meats such as fish and chicken, whole grains and no junk food.

That is to say, Dr. Eaton prescribes a diet based upon the one our hunting and foraging forebears thrived on for thousands of centuries—very low in fat (especially in saturated fat), very high in fiber, very low in salt and devoid of sugar. For its antiquity, Dr. Eaton's diet is remarkably similar to those touted today. It differs mostly by a matter of degree. For example, the diet suggested by today's medical establishment limits fat consumption to keep blood cholesterol under 200. Dr. Eaton, who considers this figure "rather high," would limit fats even more to keep cholesterol under 150. That level, he says, is a proper target. (His is 140.)

THE STONE AGE PHYSIQUE

Will we all resemble Fred Flintstone on the Stone Age Diet? In reality, prehistoric (preagriculture) peoples were tall, muscular and extremely fit—"much like today's decathlon athletes," says Dr. Eaton. They also might have lived longer lives than we do today were it not for infections, wild beasts and club blows to the head (all conditions we now have relatively under control).

Of course, our ancient ancestors' good health was attributable to more than diet: They neither drank nor smoked, and all that hunting and foraging was terrific outdoor exercise.

There's nothing wrong with meat, says Dr. S. Boyd Eaton, advocate of the Stone Age Diet. Our ancestors ate lots of it. But when they did their "shopping"—as illustrated in this cave drawing—they walked away with only the extra-lean meat of wild game. Dr. Eaton says you can find equally fat-free meat in today's supermarket if you look in the fish and poultry sections.

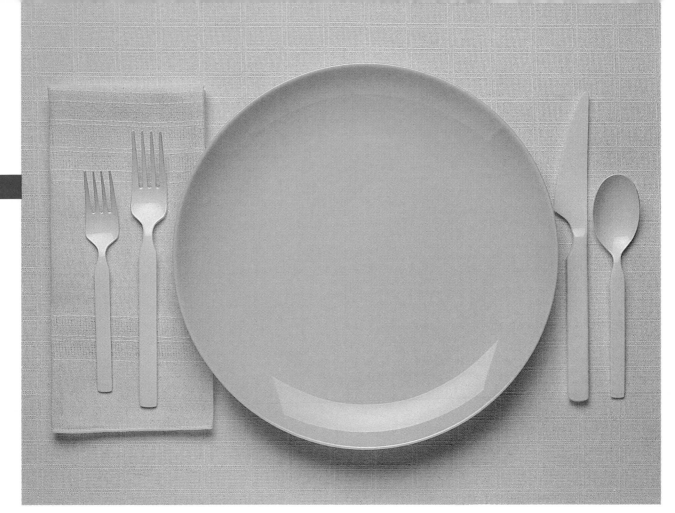

THE ULTIMATE DIET

Here's one diet that couldn't be any simpler to follow. There's no need to worry about fats, fiber, carbohydrates, cholesterol, nightshades, colorings, salicylates, yins or yangs. It doesn't matter how you eat, or when you eat. Because you *don't* eat.

"People have been fasting almost as long as they have been eating," says Allan Cott, M.D., a noted champion of the virtues of food deprivation. He strongly believes that fasting—as the title of his book *Fasting: The Ultimate Diet* indicates—is the answer to many a modern-day problem. What will fasting do for you? Just for starters, Dr. Cott says you can lose weight quickly and easily, feel better physically and mentally, look and feel younger, lower your blood pressure and cholesterol levels, get more out of sex, relieve tension, sleep better and even slow the aging process.

"Too many of us live in a limbo where we feel just 'so-so' or 'okay.' Fasting delineates the difference between feeling 'just okay' and feeling abundantly alive," says Dr. Cott.

For most of us, Dr. Cott says an occasional fast of a day or two should be enough to charge our spirits and refresh our tired bodies. Longer fasts, of

Abracadabra. Will disappearing meals cause your ills to vanish? Advocates of fasting say, "Yes, it's true."

up to a month, can be of enormous benefit to those suffering from specific health problems, like depression, schizophrenia and obesity, says Dr. Cott. (He himself has fasted for periods of up to five days.)

Is fasting safe? "We live in a culture that equates 'three squares a day' with the preservation of life itself," says Dr. Cott. But he insists that fasts for periods of up to a month are completely safe for most people. He highly recommends, however, that a fast of three days or more must be monitored by a physician who is knowledgeable about fasting.

Margaret Kaffouny, Ph.D., professor of nutrition at Florida State University, doesn't buy Dr. Cott's theories. "There's no evidence that a fast of one or two days will do any harm, but I wouldn't recommend anyone do it unless they know they could stand it," she says. "Me, if I don't eat breakfast, I know I can't make it through the day."

As for fasts of more than two days, Dr. Kaffouny is surprised that anyone would even suggest such a thing. "The evidence clearly shows that the body is worse off for it."

GOUT

In days of old, when men were bold—a gout attack could stop 'em cold. A royal pain of a disease, gout throughout history has made mincemeat of many a king and other courtly sorts—from Henry VIII to Benjamin Franklin. The helpless sufferer was often depicted with a bulbous big toe, gout's frequent foothold, propped up on a stool. Luxuriant lifestyles—rich food and drink in particular—were to blame, some have claimed. A joint of beef washed down with a flagon of claret—*that* was the culprit!

Not so, or at least not directly. As modern medicine now knows, gout is one of the most intensely inflammatory and painful forms of arthritis. About 1 percent of the U.S. population—not too many monarchs but lots of middle-aged men and some postmenopausal women—get it.

Gout announces its arrival with inflammation and throbbing pain in one of the joints. The source of this pain is the prickly movement of needlelike crystals lodged in the joints. These microscopic meddlers are solidified uric acid, a normal body substance that some gout sufferers amass at abnormally high levels.

Life is a bowl of cherries, some gout sufferers say, since adding the fruit to their daily diet. Unscientific though they may be, believers claim to have found great relief with this folk remedy.

EAT, DRINK, BUT BE WARY

For those with this particular body chemistry, certain foods—namely, those that turn into uric acid in the blood—can result in gout.

"Foods that are high in purines contribute to a higher uric acid level," says Robert Wortman, M.D., an associate professor in the Rheumatology Division of the Medical College of Wisconsin. "Foods with the highest levels are things like sweetbreads, liver, kidney and anchovies—foods more common to an 18th-century than a present-day diet."

Still, plenty of high-purine foods appear on the modern-day plate. Mincemeat and mackerel, kidney and consommé can all be dietary time bombs for the gouty.

"It's worthwhile to restrict those foods that are high in purines. This helps regulate the uric acid pool," says Charles Tourtellotte, M.D., chief of rheumatology at Temple University Hospital and Medical School.

You needn't take a puritanical approach, however, to purines. True, some high-purine foods are best avoided altogether. But a daily serving of others is quite all right. Refer to the box "Purine Sources" on page 75 to plan your pain-free menus.

Another party to gout is the beverage of choice at many a Friday night happy hour. "Alcohol and especially alcoholic binges have long been associated with gout," says Dr. Tourtellotte. Like high-purine foods, alcohol contributes to high body levels of uric acid.

THE DIETER'S DILEMMA

"The biggest problem for people with gout is being overweight," says Dr. Wortman. Heavier people tend to have high uric acid levels and high blood pressure.

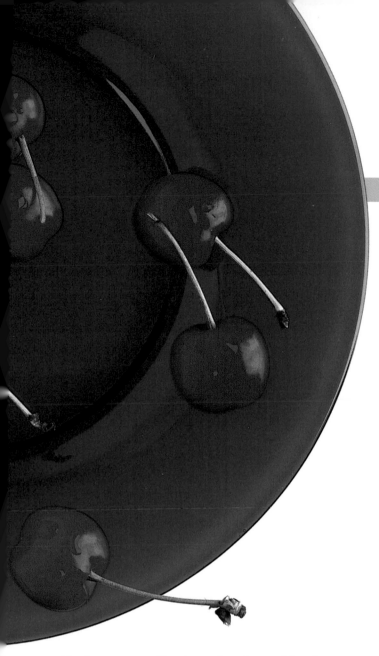

PURINE SOURCES

Foods Likely to Induce Gout Attacks (avoid at all times)

Approximate purine content ranges from 150 to 1,000 milligrams each per 3½-ounce serving.

Anchovies
Brains
Consommé
Gravies
Heart
Herring
Kidney
Liver
Meat extracts
Mincemeat
Mussels
Sardines
Sweetbreads

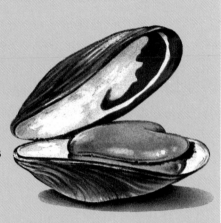

Foods That May Contribute to Gout (limit to just one serving daily)

Approximate purine content ranges from 50 to 150 milligrams each per 3½-ounce serving.

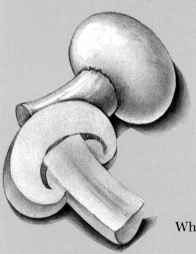

Asparagus
Beans, dry
Cauliflower
Fish*
Lentils
Meats*
Mushrooms
Oatmeal
Peas, dry
Poultry*
Shellfish
Spinach
Whole grain cereals and breads
Yeast

*Limit meat, fish or fowl to one 3-ounce serving, five days a week.

(And many medications that lower blood pressure also elevate uric acid levels.)

Having a lean body reduces the likelihood of getting gout. So one should lose weight fast, right? Wrong, because some diets can actually make things worse.

"When obese people don't eat or when they go on fasts, they metabolize their fat. That increases tissue levels of uric acid," says Dr. Tourtellotte.

The overweight person should try to slim down, but very slowly and deliberately, Dr. Tourtellotte says. Crash diets are absolutely out.

"Maintaining good health habits in general is most important," says Dr. Wortman. "Avoid excess alcohol, maintain normal body weight and try to keep your blood pressure within the normal range."

Henry VIII might have given his kingdom for some of this advice. Or at least a knighthood or two.

HEADACHES

As a researcher [someone who conducts scientific studies], I have some doubts about the relationship of diets to headaches," says Seymour Diamond, M.D., founder of the Diamond Headache Clinic and the National Headache Foundation. "As a clinician [someone who sees patients], I have no doubts." That doesn't mean a diet remedy will definitely work for you. But eliminating one or more of the foods mentioned in this section may eliminate your headache, too.

THE HOT DOG HEADACHE

The culprit isn't that familiar cuisine de ballpark per se, it's the nitrites used in the curing process. Nitrites are found in everything from luncheon meat to bacon, and there is a cure for this cure. Just add cured meats to your "foods to avoid" list.

THE ICE CREAM HEADACHE

Exactly what causes an ice cream headache isn't known. But, according to Dr. Diamond, the pain may be a response of the warm tissues of the mouth to the cold substance. Two nerves there carry impulses—including pain—to the head, which explains why the headache is generalized in the head and throat. To avoid the headache, allow small amounts of ice cream to melt or warm up in the mouth so that the mouth cools slowly.

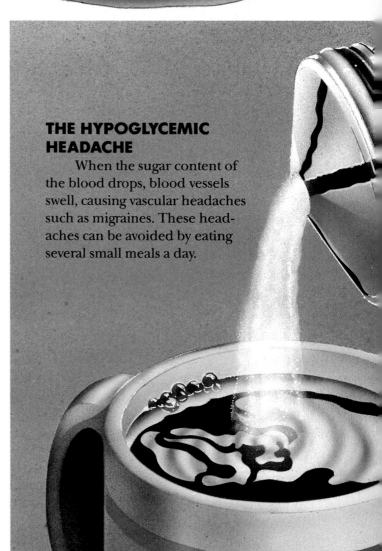

THE HYPOGLYCEMIC HEADACHE

When the sugar content of the blood drops, blood vessels swell, causing vascular headaches such as migraines. These headaches can be avoided by eating several small meals a day.

THE SALT HEADACHE

"Salt affects the blood vessels in such a way as to make you very susceptible to other substances," says John Brainard, M.D., author of *Control of Migraines.* "When the salt hits the stomach lining, it stimulates the vagus nerve, which carries the impulse to the head, causing a headache."

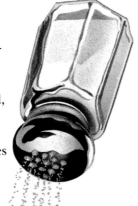

THE HANGOVER HEADACHE

This one is completely avoidable. Simply don't drink to excess. But if you expect to overindulge, says Dr. Diamond, there is a way to lessen the pain. Eating fruit or honey, even drinking tomato juice before you go out on the town, can reduce the impact of a hangover headache. Fructose helps the body metabolize ethyl alcohol, he says.

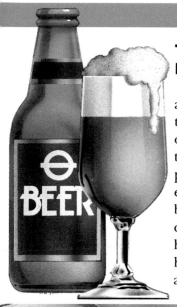

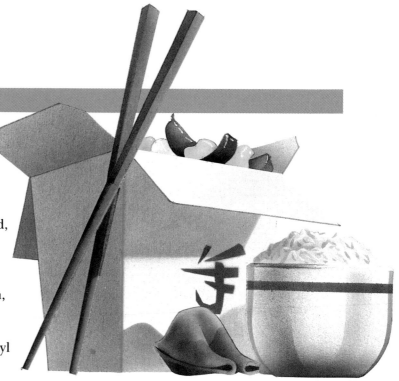

THE CHINESE RESTAURANT SYNDROME HEADACHE

Do you get headaches after eating Chinese food? It's not the Moo Goo Gai Pan but the monosodium glutamate, or MSG, that triggers this reaction. MSG headaches are most pronounced if you eat on an empty stomach, so before your Chinese dinner, eat a roll or a salad.

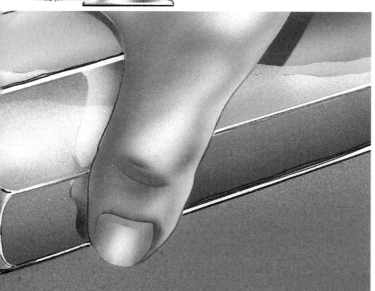

THE CAFFEINE HEADACHE

Caffeine is a vasoconstrictor—it makes your blood vessels contract. They can adapt quite readily to this semiconstricted state if you're a habitual caffeine drinker. Going cold turkey will cause the vessels to swell, leaving you with a dull withdrawal headache.

FOODS FOR THE HEADACHE-PRONE

The following foods seem relatively safe for most headache sufferers.

Dairy products: cottage cheese, cream cheese and yogurt.

Fruits: apples, apricots, bananas, blueberries, cherries and citrus fruits.

Meat: beef, chicken, duck, lamb, turkey and veal.

Vegetables: artichokes, broccoli, carrots, celery, green beans, leafy greens, mushrooms, peas and potatoes.

HEART DISEASE

It is a disease of years—years of eating the wrong foods, years of not exercising and years of microscopic, hidden changes occurring within the most remote corners of your body. As the disease progresses, the changes grow from small to large. Cholesterol, fat and calcium collect in clumps until a clogged vessel blocks blood and oxygen needed by the heart. Then the worst occurs—a heart attack.

Twenty years ago, most physicians would have said there was nothing you could do to prevent an attack. Heart disease, it seemed, just happened to some people, and if you were one of them—well, tough luck, buddy, and good luck in surgery.

But that was then. The consensus today is absolutely different: Heart disease is not only treatable, it's preventable—a disease, in fact, that can often be avoided by simple, nonmedical changes in lifestyle. One of the most important of those changes is your diet—the food you choose to put on your table.

"Diet is the cornerstone of therapy, really," says Robert Levy, M.D., cardiologist, former professor of medicine at the Columbia University College of Physicians and Surgeons in New York City, and currently president of Sandoz Research Institute, East Hanover, New Jersey.

"If there were a greater focus on nutrition, especially in the early years of life, we'd all probably get by with fewer drugs and we'd need them a lot later in life," he says.

Brian L. G. Morgan, Ph.D, acting director of the Institute of Human Nutrition at Columbia University, agrees. "Foods can't be used to cure most major diseases, but they can be very important in *preventing* a wide range of them," he says. "The high-fat diet is one obvious example: It puts you at high risk for cancer *and* heart disease. A diet low in saturated fats, on the other hand, will reduce your risk of heart disease significantly."

"Saturated fat raises your blood cholesterol more than anything else you eat," the government's National Cholesterol Education Program says in its guidelines for the public.

The right diet may accomplish more than just cutting your risk. Research out of the University of Southern California Medical School indicates that eating right can in many cases stop—and in some cases actually *reverse*—atherosclerosis, one of the main causes of heart disease.

"This study demonstrates that we now have the wherewithal to turn heart disease around in its early stages," says David H. Blankenhorn, M.D., chief investigator of the study.

THE LAZY MAN'S GUIDE TO LEAN CUISINE

So what constitutes the right diet? How, in other words, do you get the fat and cholesterol out of *your* food? The National Cholesterol Education Program offers the following suggestions to help you make your diet heart healthy and nutritionally sound:
• Use only lean meat—chicken, turkey and cuts of red meat like sirloin tip, round steak, rump roast, center-cut ham, lamb chops and tenderloin. Trim away fat before cooking the meat. You don't have to

CRACKDOWN ON COCONUT

Coconut. Mention it to most of us and we're immediately awash in a flood of Polynesian images—palms swaying under blue sky, girls in grass skirts walking on white sand beaches.

But mention it to a nutritionist and a whole different slide show goes up on the screen—one full of clogged arteries and damaged hearts.

Why? Simply because coconut oil—strangely unlike most vegetable oils—is an enormously concentrated source of saturated fats. Roughly 50 percent of the fat in butter, for example, is saturated. In coconut oil, it's a whopping 87 percent.

The message here, given that saturated fats drive your cholesterol up more than anything else? Coconut oil should be avoided.

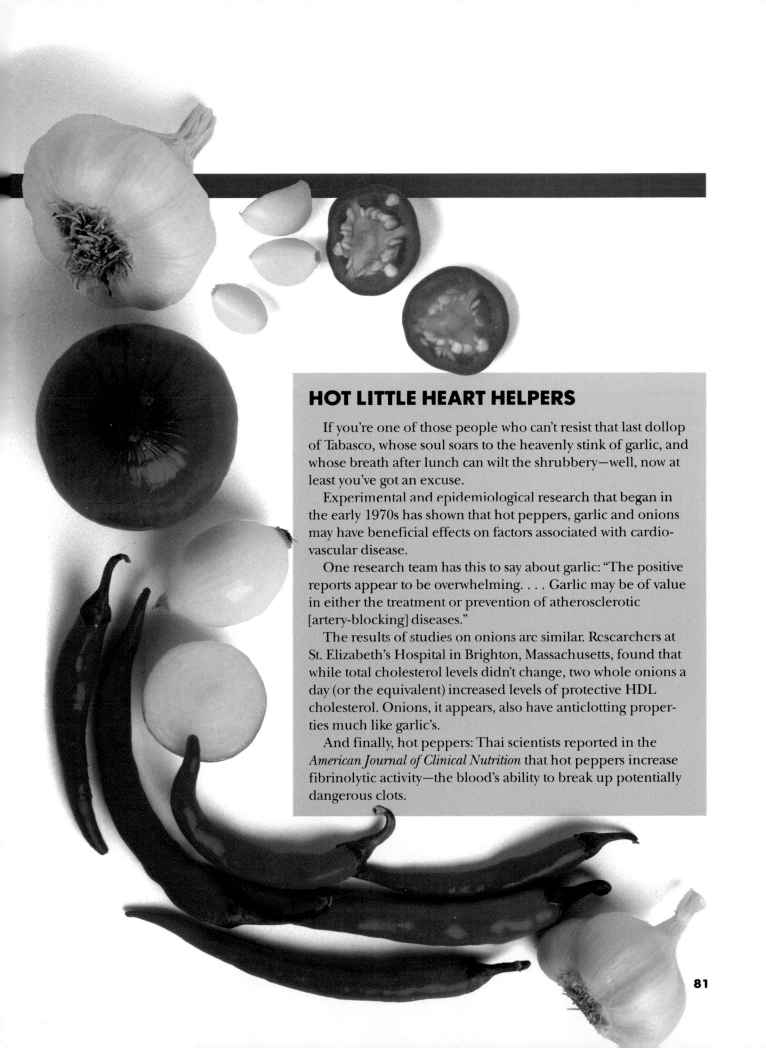

HOT LITTLE HEART HELPERS

If you're one of those people who can't resist that last dollop of Tabasco, whose soul soars to the heavenly stink of garlic, and whose breath after lunch can wilt the shrubbery—well, now at least you've got an excuse.

Experimental and epidemiological research that began in the early 1970s has shown that hot peppers, garlic and onions may have beneficial effects on factors associated with cardio-vascular disease.

One research team has this to say about garlic: "The positive reports appear to be overwhelming. . . . Garlic may be of value in either the treatment or prevention of atherosclerotic [artery-blocking] diseases."

The results of studies on onions are similar. Researchers at St. Elizabeth's Hospital in Brighton, Massachusetts, found that while total cholesterol levels didn't change, two whole onions a day (or the equivalent) increased levels of protective HDL cholesterol. Onions, it appears, also have anticlotting proper-ties much like garlic's.

And finally, hot peppers: Thai scientists reported in the *American Journal of Clinical Nutrition* that hot peppers increase fibrinolytic activity—the blood's ability to break up potentially dangerous clots.

cut down drastically on red meat; in fact, women of childbearing age who do so could risk iron-deficiency anemia.

• Eat very little high-fat, processed meat (bacon and sausage). The program says they're not particularly rich in nutrients and contain a lot of hidden fat.

• Limit organ meats—things like kidney and liver.

They are very rich in exactly what you don't want—cholesterol.

• Don't serve poultry—chicken and turkey—in fat-rich sauces, and don't fry them in oils high in saturated fats. Remove the skin and underlying fat.

• Fish, too, shouldn't be fried in saturated fats or covered with high-fat sauces.

RATING THE FATS

The Connor Cholesterol/Saturated Fat Index (CSI) makes it easy to select foods that are low in *both* cholesterol and saturated fats. The lower the CSI number, the healthier the food.

FROZEN DESSERTS (1 cup)	CSI	CALORIES
Ice milk	6	214
Sorbet	0	245
Ice cream	13	272
Sherbet	2	290
Specialty ice cream	34	684

FATS (¼ cup)	CSI	CALORIES
Peanut butter	5	353
Butter	37	430
Mayonnaise	10	431
Soft margarines	10	432
Stick margarines	15	432
Cocoa butter	47	530
Soft shortening	16	530
Vegetable oils	8	530
Bacon grease	23	541

POULTRY AND RED MEAT (3½ oz.)	CSI	CALORIES
Poultry, no skin	6	171
Beef, pork, lamb		
10% fat ground sirloin	9	214
15% fat ground round	10	258
20% fat ground chuck	13	286
30% fat ground beef	18	381
30% fat pork	18	381
30% fat lamb chops	18	381

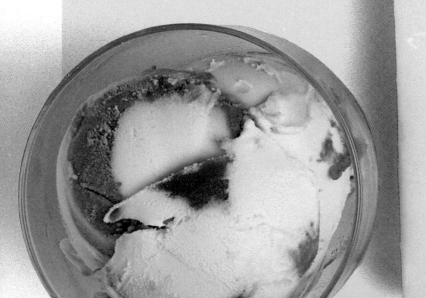

- "A reasonable approach to meat consumption," the Cholesterol Education Program says, "is to limit intake of lean meat, chicken, turkey and fish to 6 ounces per day."
- Substitute skim or low-fat (up to 1 percent) milk for whole milk, which is roughly 4 percent fat by weight. Cut back on natural and processed cheeses, switching to low-fat varieties like cottage cheese. To make sure you get enough calcium, eat at least two servings daily of very low-fat dairy products.
- Reduce your intake of fats and oils that are high in saturated fatty acids and cholesterol. Butterfat, the Cholesterol Education Program says, is your worst enemy here—to be reduced "as much as possible."

CHEESE (3½ oz.)	CSI	CALORIES
Low-fat cottage cheese	1	98
Tofu	1	98
Cottage cheese	6	139
Skim mozzarella	12	256
Cheezola	6	317
Cheddar, Swiss	26	386
Roquefort, brie	26	386

MILK PRODUCTS (1 cup)	CSI	CALORIES
Skim milk	1	88
Skim milk yogurt	1	88
1% milk	2	115
2% milk	4	144
2% plain low-fat yogurt	4	144
Milk	7	159
Liquid nondairy creamer	4	326
Sour cream	37	468
Imitation sour cream	43	499

FISH (3½ oz.)	CSI	CALORIES
Whitefish	4	91
Clams, oysters, scallops	4	91
Shrimp, crab, lobster	6	104
Salmon	5	149

EGGS	CSI	CALORIES
Whites (3)	0	51
Egg substitute (2 eggs)	1	91
Whole (2)	29	163

And instead of butter itself, try to use margarine.

• Watch labels. The Cholesterol Education Program says that palm and coconut oils, both high in saturated fats, are used regularly in baked goods, nondairy creamers, processed foods and popcorn oil. Read the labels carefully to avoid them.

• Unsaturated vegetable oils and fat don't raise blood cholesterol but are high in calories. Limit your consumption to no more than 6 to 8 teaspoons a day. Oils that the Cholesterol Education Program approves of include corn, cottonseed, olive, soybean, sunflower, safflower and rapeseed oil.

• Keep track of your egg intake. The Cholesterol Education Program says that if you eat, say, three a week, cutting down to just one is better. Egg whites, however, are cholesterol free and can be consumed freely.

• Eat plenty of fruits and vegetables. For dessert, eat fruits, low-fat yogurt and fruit ices.

• Limit fried foods and avoid frying in saturated fat (butter, lard, etc.). Good cooking methods include steaming, baking, broiling, grilling or stir-frying in small amounts of fat. You can cook foods in a microwave or in a nonstick pan without added fats.

• Chill soups after preparation. Fat will congeal on top after several hours in the refrigerator. Skim it off.

• Avoid excess salt, which can drive some people's blood pressure through the roof.

• When eating out, order entrées, potatoes and vegetables without sauces or butter. When a serving of meat is bigger than a deck of cards (3 to 4 ounces), take the excess home.

FOODS THAT COMBAT CHOLESTEROL

You've done what you can to get the fat and cholesterol out of your food. Now it's time for the next step—getting the fat and cholesterol out of *you*. Exercise will certainly help, but another solid solution is just to eat the right foods—edibles that research indicates will actively drive your cholesterol levels *down*.

Fiber. Wheat bran won't do it, but foods containing water-soluble fiber—the list includes oats, barley, fruit and beans—can reduce the cholesterol in your bloodstream by as much as *15 percent*.

"The evidence in support of fiber in general in this role isn't conclusive, but I think it's strong enough—so that a physician should advise his patients to eat more fiber as part of a heart-healthy diet," says Dr. Levy.

"Sprinkling oat bran or Metamucil on your cereal every day may only lower your cholesterol 4 or 5 percent, but that 5 percent would cut your risk of heart disease about 10 percent and could make the difference between having to take drugs and getting along without them," he says.

Guar gum. This is a common food additive. "In studies we've conducted, guar gum seems to significantly lower cholesterol, and other research institutions have had the same results," says John Farquhar, M.D., director of Stanford University's Center for Disease Prevention. "In fact, guar gum appears to lower cholesterol more substantially than fish oils or other dietary additives."

Olive oil. This monounsaturated oil, so common in the kitchens of Italy and other Mediterranean nations, also helps drive your cholesterol levels down. Its big advantage over polyunsaturates is that, unlike them, it doesn't reduce beneficial high-density lipoprotein (HDL) cholesterol while it's driving down the health-threatening low-density lipoprotein (LDL) cholesterol level.

"This fits very well with many epidemiological observations that we have from the Mediterranean countries, where there is a remarkable absence of cardiovascular disease," says Walter Mertz, M.D., director of the Beltsville Human Nutrition Research Center in Maryland.

Fish oils. The evidence accumulating in favor of making fish a regular part of your diet continues to grow. A review article published in the *Yale Journal of Biology and Medicine* reports that "the evidence shows that a diet rich in omega-3 fatty acids [fish oil] significantly reduces plasma cholesterol and triglyceride [another kind of blood fat] levels."

An interesting sidelight on fish oil is that in ani-

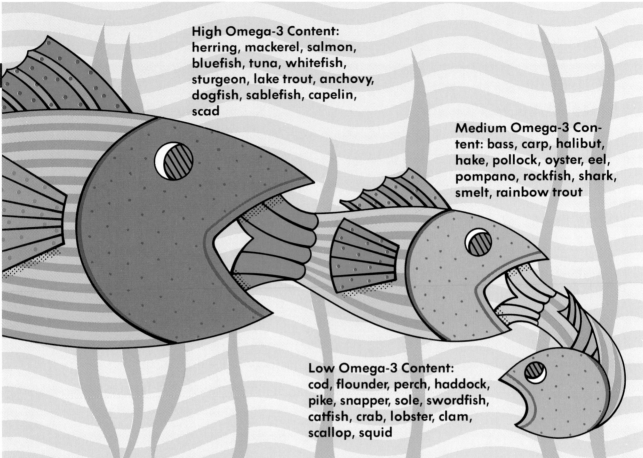

High Omega-3 Content: herring, mackerel, salmon, bluefish, tuna, whitefish, sturgeon, lake trout, anchovy, dogfish, sablefish, capelin, scad

Medium Omega-3 Content: bass, carp, halibut, hake, pollock, oyster, eel, pompano, rockfish, shark, smelt, rainbow trout

Low Omega-3 Content: cod, flounder, perch, haddock, pike, snapper, sole, swordfish, catfish, crab, lobster, clam, scallop, squid

FISHING FOR OMEGA-3

No one really knows how the omega-3 fatty acids in fish oil work. But they do work, says Brian L. G. Morgan, Ph.D., acting director of the Institute of Human Nutrition at Columbia University's College of Physicians and Surgeons.

"The research indicates that the omega-3's will increase your levels of HDL cholesterol and lower your levels of [harmful] LDL cholesterol and triglycerides," Dr. Morgan says.

"They also appear to reduce the stickiness of blood components called platelets, which may alleviate the severity of atherosclerosis. So, eating fish two or three times a week is probably a good idea. The surprising thing here is that the fatter species of fish may be better for you, since they tend to have higher levels of omega-3's."

mal studies, it significantly reduced the incidence of cancer in laboratory animals.

WHOLE FOODS, HEALTHY BODIES

The precise mechanism through which certain elements in food exert their protective effect isn't known. In this regard, Dr. Mertz offers the following caution. "There are still substances in the environment, most probably trace elements, that nutritional science hasn't recognized as important—but which nonetheless are essential.

"The point I'm making here is that, at any given time, we can never be sure that we have identified *all* the essential nutrients. And we can never be sure that if we talk about isolated nutrients (fish oil, calcium, what have you), we're giving the public what they need to know.

"Food, in other words, is always to be preferred over supplements," he says. "Let's forget about supplements, let's forget about pills—and let's realize the importance of a wholesome meal presented with variety and balance."

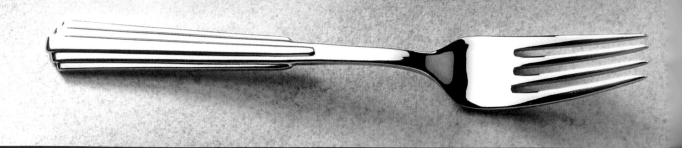

MENU MAKEOVERS

Heart boosting via your diet takes more than just cutting back on fatty meats and rich sauces. You need the know-how to make sensible choices in replacing those old mainstays with healthier alternatives. The following guide may help you understand the difference between good and bad heart-health menus.

BAD: 41 PERCENT CALORIES FROM FAT

1 cup onion soup
3½ ounces tenderloin steak, broiled
1 baked potato
1 tablespoon sour cream
½ cup green beans almandine, seasoned with salt and butter
lettuce wedge (⅙ head)
1 tablespoon Russian dressing
1 cup coffee
1 tablespoon half-and-half
1 piece pound cake

Total Calories: 876
Cholesterol: 181 milligrams

BETTER: 30 PERCENT CALORIES FROM FAT

3½ ounces baked skinless chicken breast
1 serving brown rice pilaf
½ cup steamed carrots with dill
1½ cups tossed salad (romaine, sliced mushrooms, red cabbage and sliced cucumbers)
1 tablespoon French dressing
1 whole wheat roll
1 teaspoon soft tub margarine
1 cup decaffeinated coffee
1 tablespoon 1 percent milk
1 baked apple

Total Calories: 877
Cholesterol: 93 milligrams

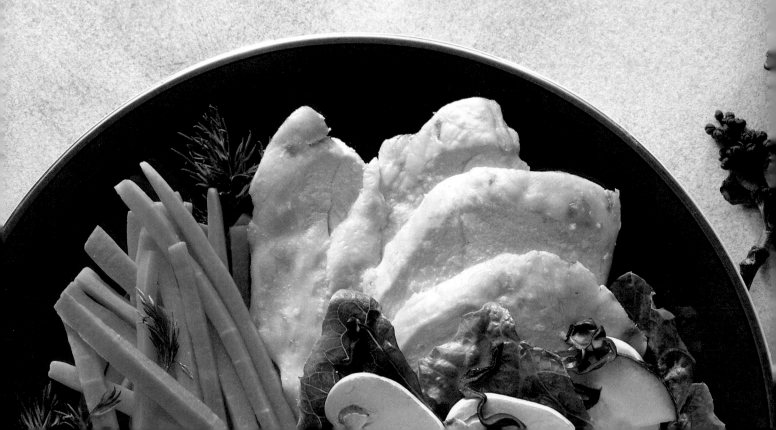

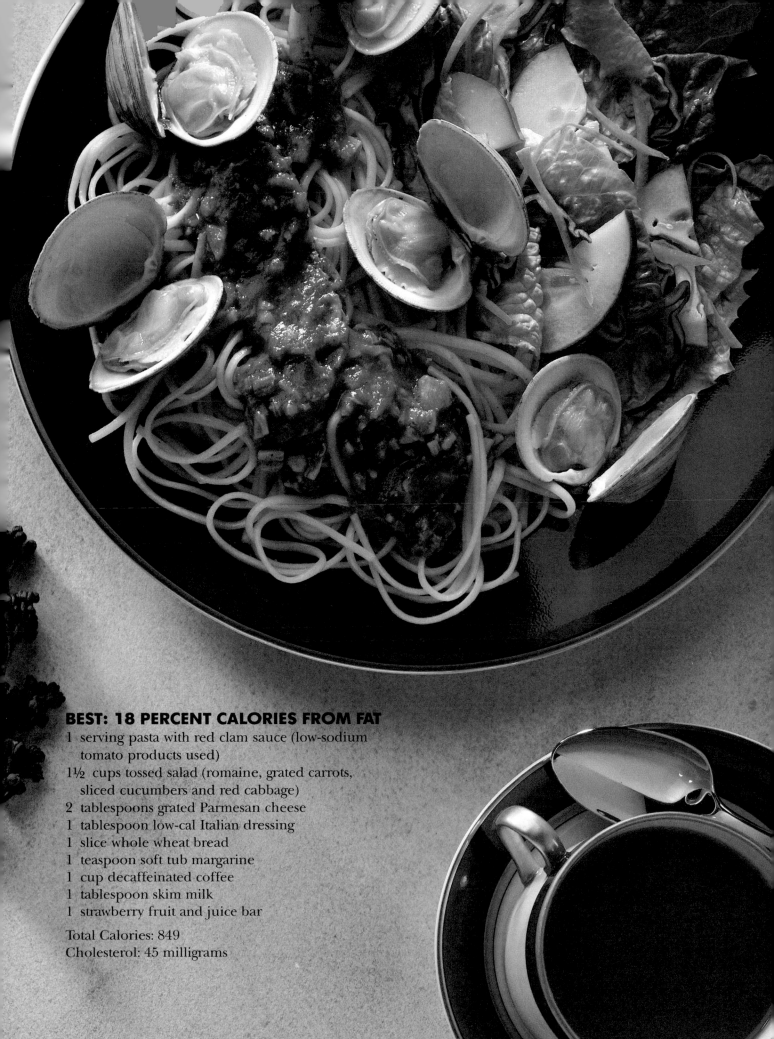

BEST: 18 PERCENT CALORIES FROM FAT

1 serving pasta with red clam sauce (low-sodium
   tomato products used)
1½ cups tossed salad (romaine, grated carrots,
   sliced cucumbers and red cabbage)
2 tablespoons grated Parmesan cheese
1 tablespoon low-cal Italian dressing
1 slice whole wheat bread
1 teaspoon soft tub margarine
1 cup decaffeinated coffee
1 tablespoon skim milk
1 strawberry fruit and juice bar

Total Calories: 849
Cholesterol: 45 milligrams

One of the ways to lower your risk of heart disease is to eat less fat—especially saturated fat. These recipes are examples of the variety of good foods that can be part of a heart-healing diet. They are low in saturated fat but offer such heart-saving elements as potassium and the monounsaturated fat in olive oil.

SIZZLED SALMON WITH CHOPPED TOMATOES AND MINT

1	lb. salmon fillet, skin removed
¼	cup orange juice
1	cup chopped tomatoes
2	Tbsp. finely minced fresh mint
	Pinch of freshly grated orange rind
2	tsp. olive oil
	Chilled orange sections, for garnish

Place salmon in a Pyrex baking dish and pour orange juice over fish. Marinate for about 10 minutes.

In a small bowl, combine tomatoes, mint and orange rind. Set aside.

Heat oil in a large, well-seasoned cast-iron skillet, or a nonstick skillet. Add salmon and orange juice and sauté until fish is sizzling and brown on the outside and cooked through, about 4 minutes on each side.

Transfer to a serving platter, top with tomato mixture and garnish with orange sections. Serve hot.

Yield: 4 servings

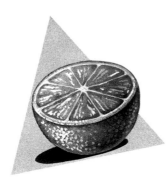

Oranges are loaded with potassium, which helps to prevent heart disease. It lowers blood pressure and counters the effects of dietary sodium.

TARRAGON CHICKEN WITH CARROTS AND LINGUINE

6	oz. uncooked linguine
1	cup stock
1	lb. skinned and boned chicken breast
1	small onion, sliced crosswise
2	carrots, cut into julienne strips
8	mushrooms, sliced
¼	cup minced fresh parsley
½	tsp. dried tarragon
	Freshly grated Parmesan cheese, for garnish
	Minced scallions, for garnish

In a large pot, cook linguine until just tender. Drain and set aside.

Pour stock into a large skillet and heat over medium heat. Cut chicken into strips 3 inches long by ½ inch wide and add to stock. Separate onion slices into individual rings and add to stock. Cook for 7 minutes, stirring frequently.

Add carrots, mushrooms, parsley and tarragon. Cook until chicken is cooked through, about 5 minutes. Add linguine to the skillet and toss to combine. Heat until linguine is hot.

Remove to a serving bowl or platter and sprinkle with cheese and scallions. Serve warm.

Yield: 4 servings

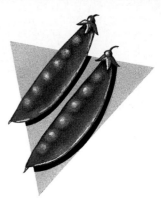

Snow peas are low in calories and fat, but fairly high in fiber—filling but not fattening.

SNOW PEAS WITH SESAME

¾	lb. snow pea pods (about 1 qt.)
1	carrot, cut into julienne strips
½	tsp. freshly grated orange rind
1	tsp. toasted sesame oil
2	tsp. toasted sesame seeds

Place pea pods and carrots in a strainer and set strainer in sink. Pour boiling water over vegetables for about 1 minute, then pat dry.

Place vegetables in a medium-size bowl and stir in orange rind, oil and seeds. Serve warm or at room temperature.

Yield: 4 servings

Sizzled Salmon with Chopped Tomatoes and Mint

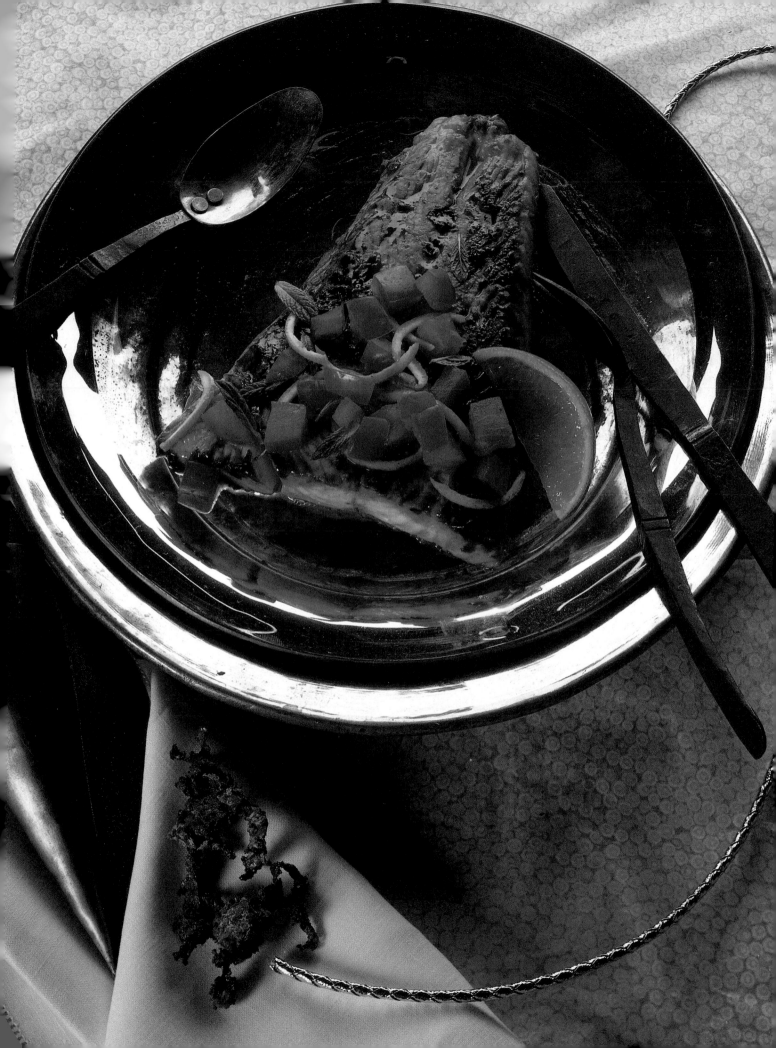

HIGH BLOOD PRESSURE

This condition works a lot like a New York City mugger. It sneaks up on you.

You go along minding your own business and then . . . BAM . . . your doctor tells you that you have hypertension and will have to take drugs for life to control your blood pressure. You probably have to go on a low-sodium diet and lose weight to boot.

That's what happens if you're lucky. Like the mugger, hypertension can kill. Untreated, it can lead to heart disease, kidney failure, strokes and even blindness.

Hypertension is also the disease that can turn some perfectly reasonable adults into irresponsible children. You know how kids don't want to take their medicine. (Aw, Mommy, do I have to?)

Many adults who feel perfectly fine even though their doctors have told them they have high blood pressure revert to that kind of behavior. They feel fine, right? So why should they have to take those bothersome and costly pills?

The good news is that in some cases they may not have to. According to a study done by researchers at Northwestern University Medical School in Chicago and the University of Minnesota and Mount Sinai Hospital in Minneapolis, treating hypertension with nutritional means rather than drugs may be "a useful first step."

The methods used in the study included a low-sodium diet, weight reduction when necessary, and cutting back on alcohol. Thirty-nine percent of those in the study who made these dietary changes were able to do without drugs during the entire four-year study. Note that these people did not go off their drugs without close supervision. If you know you have hypertension, do not try to dispense with the drugs without the help of your physician.

WAGE DIETARY WAR ON HIGH BLOOD PRESSURE

Although there is as yet no one diet to prevent or treat hypertension in everyone, experts recommend a number of dietary changes that may be of help.

Lower the boom on calories. "Of all the things

Blacks are twice as likely to get hypertension as whites, and when they do get it, they are five times as likely to get a severe form. Researchers have investigated everything from culture to diet trying to determine the reason for the difference. It may turn out to be genetic.

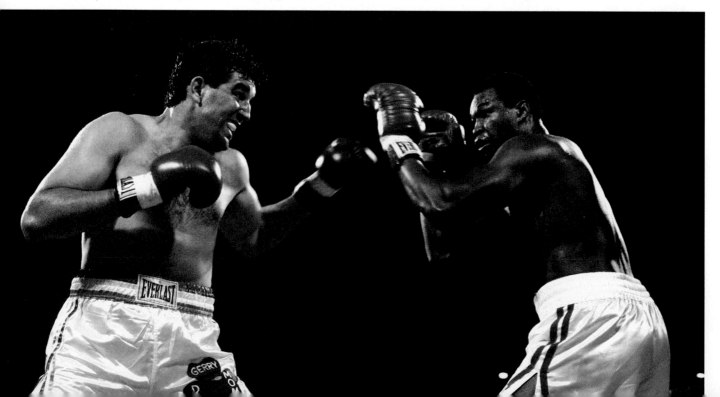

you can do, losing weight is the most important," says W. Dallas Hall, M.D., director of the Division of Hypertension at Emory School of Medicine and author of *High Blood Pressure*. "Weight loss has a beneficial effect on everyone's blood pressure, while only some people respond to reduced salt in the diet."

Of course, weight loss is only recommended for those who are 10 percent or more above their ideal weight. Weight loss will not lower your blood pressure if you are at or below that ideal.

Shake free of salt. In many cases, reducing sodium in the diet will reduce blood pressure.

Table salt is not our only source of sodium. The mineral is so all-pervasive in our diets that it is a good idea to seek professional help when going on a low-sodium diet, according to Judy Z. Miller, Ph.D., associate professor of medicine at the Hypertension Research Center, Indiana University School of Medicine. Sodium is widely used in preservatives, emulsifying agents and many other chemicals used in food processing, Dr. Miller says. A person may *think* they've cut way back on salt and still be getting much too much.

Get enough calcium and potassium. Potassium is abundant in many fruits and vegetables, including potatoes, cantaloupe, raisins and bananas. The major source of calcium is dairy products, so be careful. "So many of our dietary sources of calcium are high in fat, and people with hypertension need to reduce their intake of total fat and saturated fat," says Dr. Hall. "Use fortified skim milk."

Ban the bottle. Excessive alcohol can be a major contributor to hypertension. Allow yourself no more than two drinks a day.

Take a mackerel to dinner. Unsaturated fish oils look promising as a way of lowering blood pressure in some people. Eat more mackerel, salmon and other fish.

Have a heart. Because hyptertension is so closely related to heart disease, it is advisable to follow the dietary recommendations in the entry on heart disease, beginning on page 80.

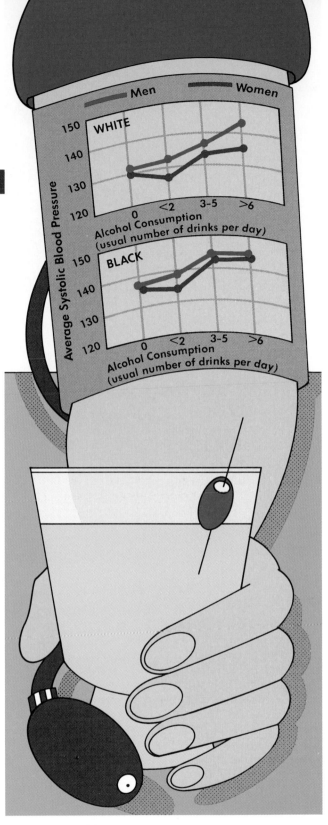

The average systolic blood pressures of both white and black women show a "J-shaped" curve. Women who drink up to two drinks a day actually have lower blood pressures than teetotalers. However, heavy drinking boosts only white people's blood pressure in a major way. Among those who consume six or more drinks a day, blood pressure levels move sharply upward, eventually meeting those of black people.

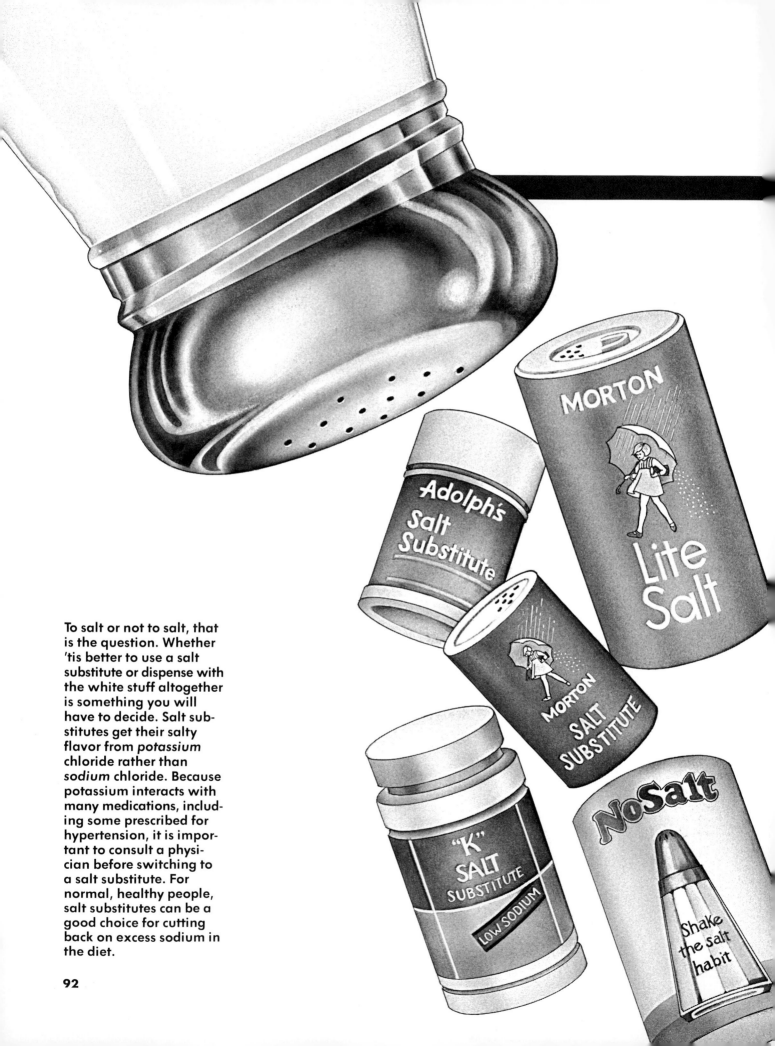

To salt or not to salt, that is the question. Whether 'tis better to use a salt substitute or dispense with the white stuff altogether is something you will have to decide. Salt substitutes get their salty flavor from *potassium* chloride rather than *sodium* chloride. Because potassium interacts with many medications, including some prescribed for hypertension, it is important to consult a physician before switching to a salt substitute. For normal, healthy people, salt substitutes can be a good choice for cutting back on excess sodium in the diet.

92

HIGH BLOOD PRESSURE
A DAY OF INTENSIVE HEALING

A.M.

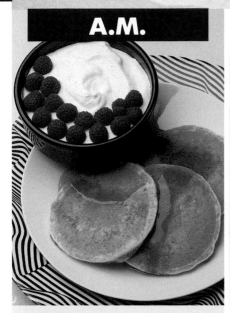

Fresh yogurt and raspberries
Whole wheat pancakes with
maple syrup
Decaffeinated coffee with
skim milk

NOON

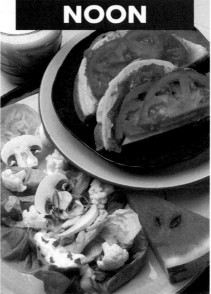

Minestrone soup
Sliced turkey, lettuce and
tomato on oatmeal
bread
Tossed salad (romaine,
lettuce, cauliflower, scallions and mushrooms)
with low-fat yogurt
dressing
Watermelon wedge
Skim milk

P.M.

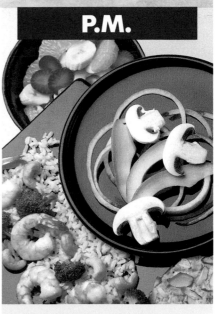

Stir-fried shrimp
Steamed brown rice
Avocado salad (avocado,
mushrooms and onions)
Fresh fruit cup (oranges,
bananas and
strawberries)

DISASTER PLATE

Slice of black olive and
anchovy double cheese
pizza
Slice of pepperoni double
cheese pizza
Beer

If you suffer from high
blood pressure, keep back.

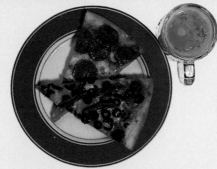

While pizza can be part of
a nutritious meal, this ver-
sion is not. The olives,
anchovies, pepperoni and
double cheese add salt
and fat, which are known
blood pressure boosters.
And so is beer—or any
other alcoholic drink.

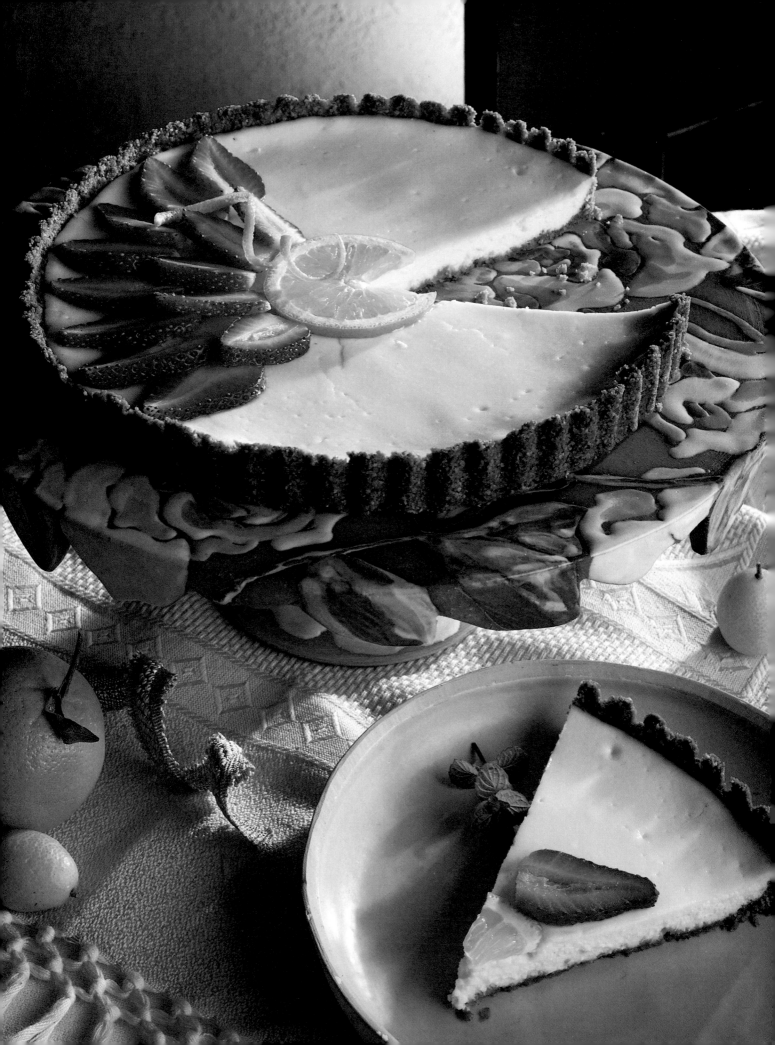

INTENSIVE HEALING RECIPES:
HIGH BLOOD PRESSURE

To control high blood pressure, it's a good idea to limit your salt and fat intake and get adequate calcium and potassium. The recipes offered here may help: cheesecake made with part-skim cheese; high-potassium avocado sauce for fish and poultry; lean London broil with a saltless marinade; and creamy, low-fat frozen yogurt.

CHEESECAKE TART

4   oz. oatmeal cookies (6 to 8 3-inch cookies)
2   Tbsp. melted sweet butter or margarine
2   cups part-skim ricotta or low-fat cottage cheese
2   egg whites
1   tsp. vanilla extract
¼   tsp. almond extract
3   Tbsp. light honey
Fresh fruit, such as tangerine or kiwi sections or berries, for garnish

Lightly oil a 9-inch tart pan that has a removable bottom.

Place cookies and butter or margarine in a food processor or blender and process until crumbly. Press mixture onto bottom and sides of tart pan, then refrigerate.

Preheat the oven to 325°F.

Place cheese, egg whites, vanilla and almond extracts and honey in the food processor or blender and process until smooth.

Spoon filling into tart shell and bake until firm, about 30 minutes. Chill and garnish with fresh fruit before serving.

Yield: 8 servings

AVOCADO SAUCE FOR FISH AND POULTRY

1   large avocado
Juice and pulp of 1 lime
Pinch of ground turmeric
Pinch of chili powder
Pinch of dried oregano
1   tsp. finely minced garlic

Peel and pit avocado and place in a food processor or blender.

Add lime, turmeric, chili powder, oregano and garlic and process until smooth. Serve with poached fish, grilled chicken or steamed prawns, or use as a binder for chicken or fish salad (which should be served immediately or it will turn dark).

Yield: 4 servings

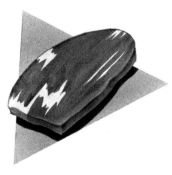

London broil is a good choice if you want to have steak for dinner. Compared to other cuts of beef, it is fairly low in fat. This 3-ounce choice top round has about 5½ grams of fat per serving, while a serving of choice flank steak has about 12 grams.

LONDON BROIL WITH NO-SALT MARINADE

12   oz. lean top round, ¾ inch thick
⅓   cup red wine vinegar
3   cloves garlic, finely minced
3   bay leaves, crushed
2   tsp. olive oil

Trim all visible fat from meat, then pierce through with a fork in about a dozen places. Place meat in a shallow baking dish or ovenproof casserole.

In a medium-size bowl, combine vinegar, garlic, bay leaves and oil. Pour mixture over meat, cover and refrigerate overnight.

Preheat the broiler. Place meat on a slotted broiler pan and broil until cooked through, about 5 minutes on each side for medium rare. Serve warm or chilled.

Yield: 4 servings

EASY FROZEN YOGURT

2   cups plain low-fat yogurt
¼   cup frozen orange juice concentrate
1   tsp. vanilla extract

In a medium-size bowl, mix all ingredients. Freeze for about 4 hours, stirring hourly for the first 3 hours.

Yield: 4 servings

Cheesecake Tart

95

IMMUNITY

Your immune system in action . . . think of it as a kind of "Cell Wars." Congress doesn't have to approve it, though, because the space it's based in is your own. "It's your self-defense system," says William Adler, M.D., chief of the Clinical Immunology Section of the National Institute on Aging.

ANOREXIA: A PUZZLE

Food for thought. That's about all anorexics do with food—they think about it. They surely don't eat much of it.

So you would think that as a group they would be likely candidates for picking up lots of infections, right? *Wrong.*

While malnourished people in general seem to be more likely than others to get infections, recent research involving anorexics found otherwise.

When Robin Wolstencroft, a researcher in the Immunology Department of the Rayne Institute, Saint Thomas' Hospital, London, studied the immune system of anorexics, he was surprised by what he found. "Our impression from the study shows that they don't seem to have exceptional problems with infections. In some immunological aspects, they are no worse off than well-nourished people."

But it's a thin line between being no worse off and having problems. Fima Lifshitz, M.D., a pediatric nutritionist at North Shore University Hospital, Manhasset, New York, found that an anorexic's weight—if it's low enough—weighs heavy on the immune system. "We studied people with a mean weight deficit of 38 percent below their normal body weight. We found that if they are severely underweight, they are more susceptible to infection."

The moral: The immune system is immune to nutritional insults—up to a point.

"It's an adaptive system," he says, "that has developed as a way of defending our bodies against foreign bacteria, viruses or other abnormal intruders."

As a defense tactic, immunity is the sum of many parts. "Your immune system has several different components," according to Brian L. G. Morgan, Ph.D., assistant professor of human nutrition at Columbia University College of Physicians and Surgeons.

"Your skin and the lining of your lungs and other organs are one part. Another line of defense includes T-cells, B-cells and the production of antibodies, which kill bacteria. And in the third line of resistance, other special cells actually engulf and then kill bacteria," he explains.

INVASION OF THE ANTIBODY SNATCHERS

Even the most well-coordinated weaponry can misfire, however, if its defenses are outflanked. And the immune system is no exception.

"Nutrition is critical," says Ranjit Kumar Chandra, M.D., professor of pediatric research, medicine and biochemistry and director of the Immunology Department, Memorial University of Newfoundland.

Dr. Chandra has been studying the role nutrition plays with the immune system for the past 15 years. He believes that "there is no doubt that moderate or even marginal deficiencies in nutrition can impair your immunity." Malnourishment is your immune system's worse enemy.

"Deficiencies in zinc, vitamin A, iron and the B-complex vitamins, especially B_6, can have profound effects on the immune system," Dr. Chandra says.

Age can also put the damper on your immune system. T-cells are important combatants in your body's fight against invading infections. But like the old missiles of the 1950s, their ability to be effective declines with age.

"With advancing years, you have fewer T-cells that can function," says Dr. Adler. "Because of that, the system is less efficient, it can't deal with infec-

THE BREASTFED ADVANTAGE

Ah, the new baby has his mother's eyes— and if he's breastfed, he may have her immunity as well. "We believe that breast milk may actually stimulate the immune system of the baby," says Ranjit Kumar Chandra, M.D.

Breast milk is loaded with IgA—a type of antibody activity, according to Dr. Chandra. Since babies don't make their own IgA, they need to get it in the breast milk. The milk coats their gastrointestinal tract with a protective coating and prevents babies from getting germs that would otherwise pass through their stomachs and into their system, perhaps resulting in allergies down the road.

For this reason, even small amounts of breast milk will go a long way in helping your baby.

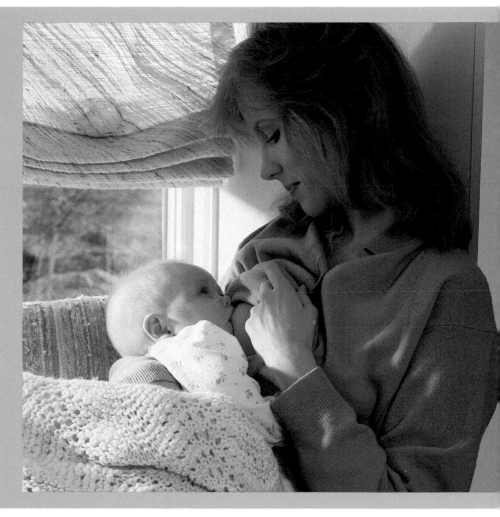

tious agents as well, and you become more susceptible to diseases."

Those T-cell missiles start rusting out a lot sooner than you may think. "The thymus, where T-cells are made, begins to atrophy after puberty," says Jeffrey Blumberg, Ph.D., assistant director of the U.S. Department of Agriculture's Human Nutrition Center at Tufts University. "The wasting away of this gland doesn't have any great functional impact at first," he says, "but by the time you reach 60 . . . bang!"

Downhill from puberty may be a hard pill to swallow, but it seems drugs can also take their toll on the immune system. "If medications that impair nutrient absorption are taken chronically, the immune system won't operate properly," cautions Dr. Morgan.

So what's the cure to shore up your defense system? Most experts agree that an increase in the amount you spend on vitamins will do little good for your total immune budget. In fact, it could be harmful.

WHEN MORE IS LESS

"Having too little of most nutrients will decrease your immunity," says Dr. Morgan. "But there's very

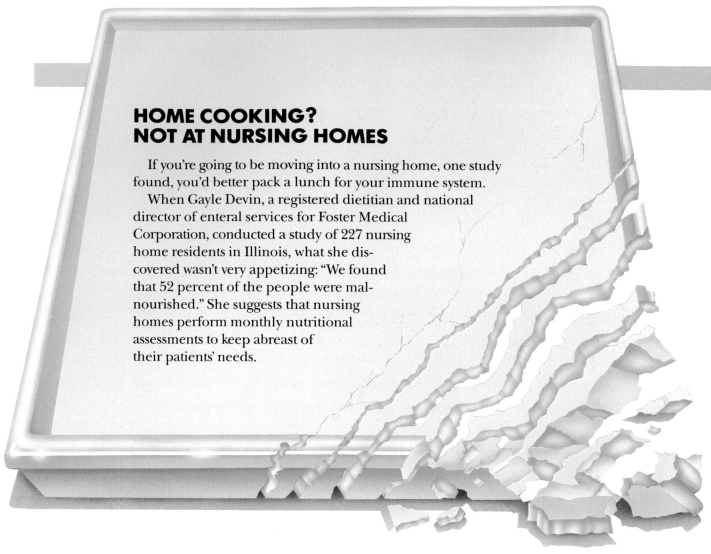

HOME COOKING?
NOT AT NURSING HOMES

If you're going to be moving into a nursing home, one study found, you'd better pack a lunch for your immune system.

When Gayle Devin, a registered dietitian and national director of enteral services for Foster Medical Corporation, conducted a study of 227 nursing home residents in Illinois, what she discovered wasn't very appetizing: "We found that 52 percent of the people were malnourished." She suggests that nursing homes perform monthly nutritional assessments to keep abreast of their patients' needs.

little evidence to show that taking more than adequate amounts of nutrients will improve your immunity."

"You can't increase your immunity beyond normal limits by what you eat," adds Dr. Chandra, "But by eating a well-balanced diet, you can keep your immune system at its optimal level."

For elderly people, a well-balanced diet is crucial. "The older you get, the better your diet should be," says Dr. Adler.

And if you want to really help your immune system when you're old, the time to do it is when you're young. "Some of the research we're doing suggests that the rate of decline of the immune response may be slowed by a well-balanced diet early on," says Dr. Blumberg. "It's not simply that you aren't eating enough of the right things when you

get older. Rather, if you had been eating enough of the right things when you were younger, the decline might not occur at such a fast rate."

So what should you eat? Research is pointing to some particular nutrients that should be at the top of your grocery list.

FUEL FOR YOUR DEFENSE SYSTEM

Dr. Morgan advises making sure that the following vitamins and minerals are amply provided.

Vitamin A. "This nutrient is involved in protein synthesis. Cells are made of protein, so if you can't produce protein, you can't make the cells you need to kill bacteria." Yellow, orange and dark green vegetables are good sources of vitamin A.

B complex. "Folate is a key to cell division; you need it to make new cells. Deficiencies in other

B vitamins lead to dry, scaly skin, sores in the mouth and on the tongue, and cracks in the corners of your mouth. All of these lesions are open to infections," says Dr. Morgan. Good sources of B vitamins include whole grains, milk, peanuts, poultry, fish, liver, fruit and raw green vegetables.

Vitamin C. "This keeps the white cells healthy so they can produce antibodies to kill bacteria," says Dr. Morgan. Look for C-rich foods like citrus fruits or raw tomatoes.

Vitamin E. "A low intake of this vitamin increases susceptibility to infection," says Dr. Morgan. In experiments with laboratory animals, adds Dr. Blumberg, "we actually got an immunostimulation with vitamin E. It optimized the vigor of the immune response."

It's found in wheat germ, green vegetables and whole grain.

Zinc. "This mineral is also needed to produce protein, but too much of it impairs the absorption of iron and other nutrients," according to Dr. Morgan. You can get safe levels by eating beef, whole wheat products and oysters.

All of the experts advise that eating foods rich in these nutrients is the best way of maintaining your immune system at its optimal level, and that overdoses of supplements may actually harm your system. Dr. Morgan emphasizes, "People need to have a really good, balanced diet. That, and possibly a daily multiple vitamin, is all most of us need to keep our immune systems functioning well."

THE PARADOX OF IRON

This bulldozer is doing to a mound of iron ore something similar to what your body does to iron when you have an infection: gets it under control.

"During an infection, the body tries to sequester iron," says Adria Rothman Sherman, Ph.D., chairperson of the Department of Home Economics at Rutgers University and a researcher who has studied the effect iron has on the immune system.

"The body tries to remove iron from easy accessibility to the infection. Just as your body needs iron, bacteria also need iron to develop. The body removes the iron from the site of the infection so that the infectious organism can't use it."

That's why you shouldn't try to iron out an infection once you've caught something, Dr. Sherman adds. "If you have an infection, I would not recommend taking iron. It's important to have it in your system before the infection to help normal cell development, but if you take it during an infection, you may

inadvertently help the bacteria grow."

To ensure an iron-rich diet, Dr. Sherman advises eating iron-rich foods like lean red meats, liver, whole wheat and fortified grain products, and leafy vegetables such as spinach.

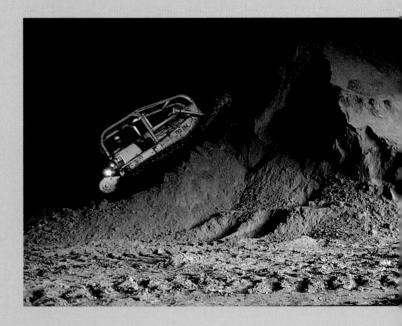

IMPOTENCE

How about a nice warm bowl of sea slug soup? Perhaps a concoction of rhinoceros horn would be more to your liking? A pinch of tiger whisker? A large lump of camel hump fat? A hearty cowboy meal of raw bull's testicles? What could possibly be the rationale for creating such nauseating dishes? The answer is S-E-X.

For centuries, the kitchen has been the site of a curious kind of foreplay. But if you ask a urologist or a sex therapist about aphrodisiacs, they will tell you that there's no such animal. Or vegetable.

But (and this is a big but) there *is* a whole lot you can do in the kitchen to prevent impotence.

According to Adrian Zorgniotti, M.D., urolo-

THE TREE OF LIFE

Time was when you could find the bark of the African yohimbe tree in the herb section of your local health food store and brew yourself a cup of tea. It was also available as a street drug, known for a while as "yo yo."

The attraction? It seems the stuff was supposed to be an aphrodisiac. Sip some tea or pop a pill and *Wow!* instant lust. Finished laughing yet? It seems that yohimbe really works. Sometimes. Yohimbine, the active ingredient of the bark, has been synthesized and is coming under serious scientific scrutiny.

Kelly Reid of the Department of Psychology, Queens University, Ontario, along with James Owen, Ph.D., pharmacologist with the Kingston Psychiatric Hospital, also in Ontario, recently participated in a study of the drug in which half the impotent men in the study noticed an improvement, and among that fortunate group half experienced a complete return to normal function.

Available only by prescription in the United States, yohimbine can produce dangerous side effects, including high blood pressure.

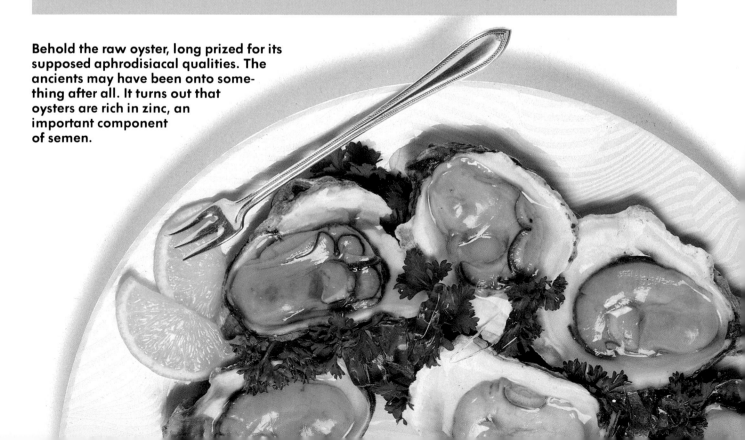

Behold the raw oyster, long prized for its supposed aphrodisiacal qualities. The ancients may have been onto something after all. It turns out that oysters are rich in zinc, an important component of semen.

gist and president of the International Society for Impotence Research, most impotence is really a blood flow problem. A man suffers hardening of the arteries in the penis for the same reasons he suffers heart disease.

"Of course, it's primarily used to treat heart disease, but any good cholesterol-reducing diet also would be helpful as a preventive, although it will not cure the problem," says Dr. Zorgniotti.

DR. BERGER'S LOW-FAT DIET

A man's inability to get an erection is often a physical rather than a mental problem. And often that physical problem developed gradually through years of poor dietary practices. That's the word from Richard E. Berger, M.D., urologist and coauthor of *BioPotency: A Guide to Sexual Success.*

"Diet plays as big a role or bigger in erection problems as it does in any other problem relating to blood vessels," says Dr. Berger. "In reality, the penis is a specialized blood vessel."

A study found that men with erection problems were also likely to have diabetes or high blood pressure, have high cholesterol or high triglyceride levels or be smokers. The more of these risk factors, the higher the likelihood of impotence. Another study found hardening of the arteries in the penises of men over 30.

Many of these factors are altered by diet, says Dr. Berger. He added that there is even some evidence that changes in diet can decrease vascular disease over the long haul. "I've had people say when they change their diet that they feel better and their sex lives improve." So a low-fat diet is the way to go to prevent impotence and perhaps even improve an existing problem.

As for alcohol, says Dr. Berger, it is "a direct testicular toxin. It damages the testicles as well as the liver and decreases the production of male hormone."

And you thought steak and beer were he-man fare; *au contraire.* For a romantic dinner, try a large salad and a small glass of wine.

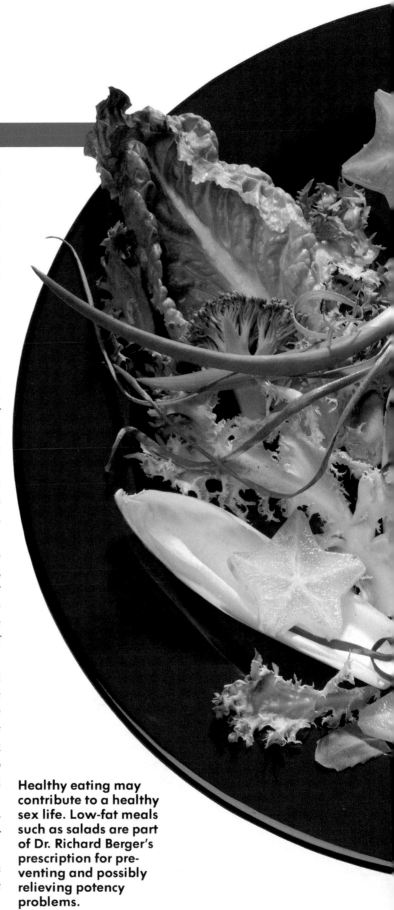

Healthy eating may contribute to a healthy sex life. Low-fat meals such as salads are part of Dr. Richard Berger's prescription for preventing and possibly relieving potency problems.

INDIGESTION

Let them laugh. *They* never had to pace the floor at night because lying down brings on the pain. The folks who snicker over television's antacid commercials don't know just how bad it can hurt.

Okay, so maybe it *is* a little funny when feeding too freely at the trough of human indulgence results in a bout of blazing tummy. That, after all, is a clear case of cosmic retribution for too much turkey stuffing and mincemeat pie.

But what about the poor soul who suffers day in and day out?

The American Digestive Disease Society operates a public information service known as Gutline. Executive director Martin Hassner says that 98 percent of the calls for help come from people suffering from *chronic* digestive problems. Some of them have experienced heartburn so intense that they've landed in the emergency ward under the mistaken impression that they were having a heart attack. Those people weren't laughing.

GET TO THE ROOT OF THE PAIN

That brings us to something important that needs to be said before we can talk about food.

All kinds of symptoms, everything from heartburn to that bloated, wish-I-hadn't-eaten-that feeling, get labeled as "indigestion." The symptoms can mean that you ate a food that just didn't sit well with you or they can be a signal that something serious is wrong.

The nerves of the chest and abdominal cavity are so crisscrossed that some pretty serious conditions can masquerade as plain old "indigestion," says Donald Henderson, M.D., of the West Gastroenterology Group in Los Angeles.

So don't play dietary roulette looking for the miraculous combination of foods that is going to make you feel better. If your pain and discomfort come back over and over again, or if your pain is severe enough to keep you from functioning normally, it is time to see a physician.

"The intestinal tract is really a wonderful system.

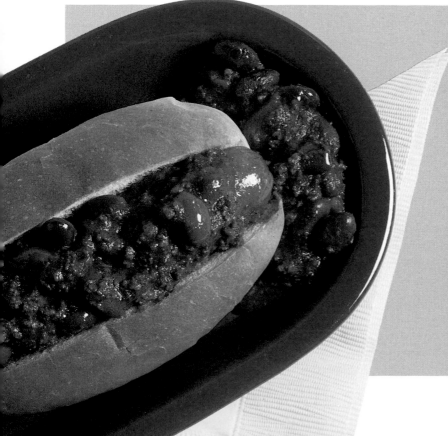

TAME THOSE BEANS

Wash the gas right out of those beans.

You keep hearing that beans are a good fiber food, full of protein and low in fat, and you wonder how anything so good for you can make you feel *so-o-o-o* uncomfortable.

If beans give you gas, a little kitchen trickery might enable you to enjoy them after all.

Soak beans in water for three to four hours. After soaking, change the water and boil the beans for 30 minutes. Then discard the water. If the beans require more cooking, again use fresh water.

You might wash quite a few nutrients down the drain, but you're also flushing away the flatulence factor.

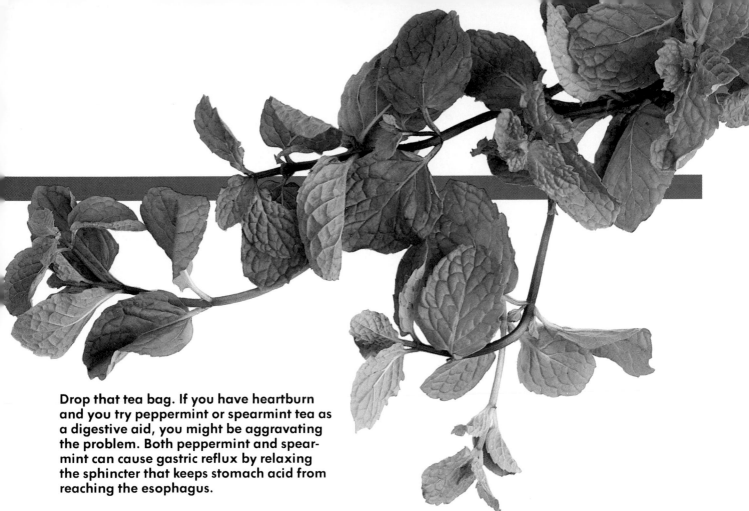

Drop that tea bag. If you have heartburn and you try peppermint or spearmint tea as a digestive aid, you might be aggravating the problem. Both peppermint and spearmint can cause gastric reflux by relaxing the sphincter that keeps stomach acid from reaching the esophagus.

It adapts to many different changes of diet, whether it's alcohol or Mexican food or whale blubber," says Dr. Henderson. "How we eat, or eating to excess, is usually more of a factor than what we eat."

Those occasional bouts of discomfort that *are* food-related indigestion can usually be traced to either heartburn or excess gas.

PUT OUT THE FLAMES

Feel like your chest is on fire when heartburn flares up? That could be because something is really burning—your esophagus, to be precise. Heartburn happens when the acid contents of the stomach end up where they aren't supposed to be (gastric reflux).

The lower esophageal sphincter, or LES, is like a door between your stomach and your esophagus. When you're not actually eating, the LES is supposed to remain closed tightly like a fist. But, if some of the acid gets through the LES and ends up in your esophagus, it causes a burning sensation. Oh, boy, does it burn.

You don't have to just lie there and stew in your own juices, however. There are a number of things you can do to prevent that gastric fire.

Eat less fat. Fatty meals are harder to digest and remain in the stomach longer.

Eliminate problem foods. Some substances actually cause the LES to relax, which in turn makes it easier for stomach acid to flow up into your esophagus. The worst offenders are coffee (including decaffeinated), peppermint, spearmint, alcohol and chocolate.

Think small. Smaller, more frequent meals may help.

Think empty. If nighttime heartburn is a problem, don't consume food or drink for three to six hours before going to bed.

Watch those combinations. Many medications, particularly pain medications, increase the stomach's acid response to foods. You might find that hot, spicy foods which don't normally bother you might suddenly become a problem if you've taken an aspirin.

DEFLATE THAT GAS PROBLEM

Most stomach and intestinal gas doesn't come from food at all.

"Beans, onions, hot tamales—the intestinal tract can adjust to all those things by and large," says Dr. Henderson. "Actually, swallowed air is responsible for 80 to 90 percent of gas. Food accounts for only 20 percent."

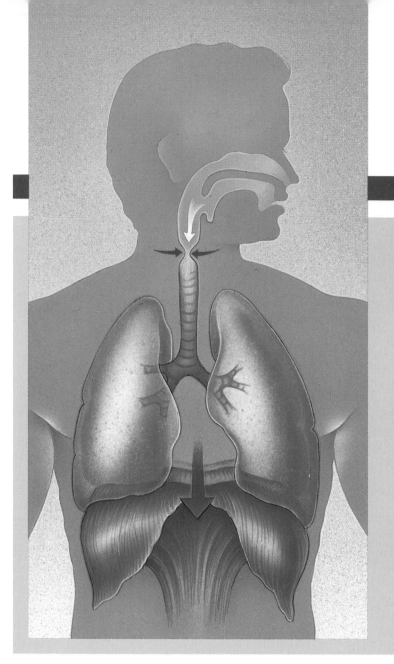

HOW DO YOU HIC?

So, besides being something that makes you feel silly, what exactly is a hiccup?

A hiccup is . . . a disagreement, a family quarrel if you will, between your diaphragm and your voice box.

When the nerves that control your diaphragm are irritated, let's say by a cold drink gulped too quickly, they trigger an involuntary spasm. The spasm of the diaphragm causes a quick intake of air.

Now if that was all there was to it, you would gasp and that would be the end of it. But no, the voice box gets into the act. As the air is sucked in, the voice box and vocal cords, known as the glottis, snap closed and prevent the breath from entering.

Your diaphragm says "yes" to taking a breath; your glottis says, "no." And you say, "HIC!"

People sometimes gulp air when they eat under stress. So avoid emotional upsets at the table. It's also a good idea to eat more slowly.

But if your problem *is* food, it may be hard to isolate the culprit. Our digestive systems are highly individualized. Foods that cause problems for one person may be perfectly all right for another. You need to be something of a sleuth to figure out which foods are troublesome for you personally. There are, however, a few foods that tend to cause problems for a large number of people.

One of those is milk. You might wonder how the number one best food for infants could be pure agony for so many adults. But as they grow up, some people lose the means to digest dairy products. Any time they eat dishes that contain large amounts of milk or cheese, they are going to feel just plain lousy.

If you suspect this might be your problem, see the entry on lactose intolerance, beginning on page 110.

THE FIBER CHALLENGE

High-fiber foods also tend to cause increased intestinal gas. If you are trying to switch to a healthier diet, that can present a real problem.

Well, hang in there. Your digestive system can and will adjust to more fiber if you'll just give it time, says Samuel Klein, M.D., assistant professor of gastroenterology at the University of Texas Medical Branch, Galveston. Usually two to three weeks is all it takes, so he advises a "slow and steady" approach.

It also helps to drink more water. Water helps relieve constipation and helps fiber move through the digestive system.

INDIGESTION
A DAY OF INTENSIVE HEALING

A.M.	NOON	P.M.

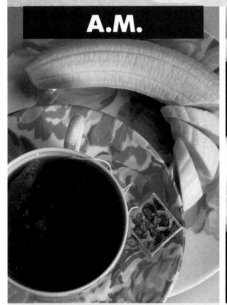 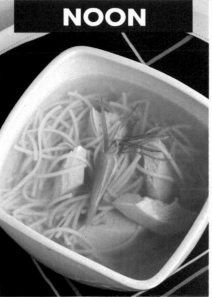 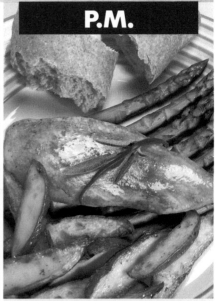

Oat bran cereal
Banana
Strawberry-leaf tea or
   Postum

Snack
Baked apple
Sweet acidophilus milk
Water

Chicken noodle soup
Salmon salad (salmon,
   romaine, lettuce, beets
   and carrots)
Water

Snack
Hummus
Pita wedges
Apple juice

Baked chicken breast
Asparagus
Roasted new potatoes
Whole wheat bread
Water

Snack
Blueberry muffin
Sliced pears, almonds and
   yogurt
Water

DISASTER PLATE

Hot Italian sausage sub
   with fried red and green
   peppers
Black coffee

   If you put all the worst
offenders of digestion into

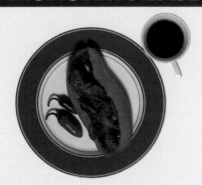

one meal, you could hardly
beat this combination. It is
high in fat, low in fiber and
it is a bit too spicy. Black
coffee, hot and acidic, adds
to the potential for tummy
trouble.

INSOMNIA

It's 3 o'clock in the morning and you still can't sleep. The dog, the kids, even the crickets outside your window long ago drifted off to dreamland, but you have entered—The Twilight Zone. You toss and turn till the sheets are in a tangle. You watch imaginary movies on the ceiling. You count sheep, count the hours till dawn, count on another groggy-eyed day ahead.

Such is the recurring nightmare of the person suffering from insomnia, a chronic difficulty with falling asleep or staying asleep. While treatment of the disorder can be complex, sleep experts are waking sufferers up to a few simple nutritional remedies that can be of help.

ELIMINATE THE NEGATIVE

For starters, "Eliminate those things likely to keep you awake," says Henry Lahmeyer, M.D., director of the sleep disorders center at the University of Illinois, Chicago.

"Alcohol is the worst offender. You have withdrawal symptoms from it in the middle of the night, and that wakes you up," Dr, Lahmeyer says. The same principle operates with the addictive nicotine in cigarettes—another good reason not to smoke.

Coffee and caffeinated tea are definite deterrents to shut-eye. Many sleep experts advise their patients to strictly avoid caffeine in the afternoon unless they want to be bright-eyed long after the sun goes down. Watch out, by the way, for caffeine in unlikely places; certain analgesics and some anti-inflammatories include the stimulant among their ingredients. Check the label before you take an anti-dozing dose.

ASSIMILATE THE POSITIVE

Laying off of sleep-inhibiting substances may be all you need to get a good night's worth of Z's. But you might need to add items to your diet as well.

"Foods rich in tryptophan can help," says Elliott Phillips, M.D., medical director of the sleep disorders center at Holy Cross Hospital in California.

Tryptophan, Dr. Phillips explains, is an amino acid that serves as a primary ingredient in the human body's production of serotonin, a chemical in the brain that appears to play an important part in normal human sleep.

"The calming chemical" is what Judith Wurtman, M.D., calls serotonin. A research scientist at the Massachusetts Institute of Technology and author of the book *Managing Your Mind and Mood through Food,* Dr. Wurtman says that feelings of stress and tension take a back seat to relaxation when your brain is actively using serotonin.

Foods high in tryptophan include milk, cheddar cheese, turkey, tuna and peanuts. But for best results, says Dr. Phillips, eat a small portion of foods high in tryptophan *along with* carbohydrates like bread or cereal. This combination helps your body assimilate the substance more efficiently.

MILK—YES OR NO?

Remember those sleepless nights as a kid when, as far as Mom was concerned, a nice glass of warm milk was just what the sandman ordered? While milk does help some people, there's no hard proof that it works, says one sleep expert. Milk *does* contain sleep-inducing tryptophan, but it also has other amino acids that compete for absorption by the brain. Still, if milk is part of a relaxing presleep ritual, it very likely will work—so drink up. And pleasant dreams!

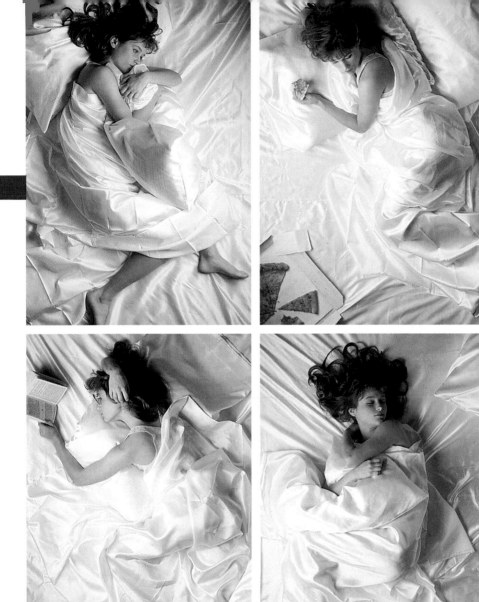

Do you have trouble sleeping? Join the club. In surveys of the general population, about one-third of the respondents had some difficulty relating to sleep. Of the various sleep disorders, insomnia is the most common and affects women and elderly persons most often.

Dr. Wurtman takes this approach a step further: To get the most tryptophan to the brain quickly, eat carbohydrates alone, without protein. "Eating carbohydrates alone has a calming, focusing effect," she says. Hence, unless you're averse to refined sugar, she advises treating yourself before bed to 1½ cups of any breakfast cereal without milk, or even a gooey Pop-Tart. (Just be sure to brush your teeth.) Fruit, by the way, won't help you sleep; your body absorbs fruit sugars too slowly. In the starch department, try a bagel, 2 ounces of dry-popped popcorn or eight triple RyKrisp crackers. By the way, these recommended amounts are for people of normal weight.

Tryptophan (available as L-tryptophan in most health food stores) is effective in supplement form as well. "Three to four 500-milligram pills can reduce

by about one-third the amount of time it takes to get to sleep," says Dr. Phillips. It is even more helpful, he says, in preventing repeated awakenings during the night. (Supplements are not recommended, however, for children, pregnant women or for people who have adrenal gland problems.)

Herbalists claim that a number of herbs may help, too. Relax before bedtime with a warm cup of spearmint, peppermint or orange bergamot mint tea. Herbalists also recommend hot teas of catnip or hops to help you sleep.

The real key to healthy sleep is to develop consistently healthy habits overall, says Dr. Phillips. "Eating regular meals at regular times of day is probably much more important than eating or not eating specific foods before bed."

WALTER KEMPNER AND THE RICE DIET

This is a monotonous diet and it does not taste good. It can never become popular. It is a disagreeable medicine. One has to eat it for quite a while before its full effect becomes apparent. . . . There is only one excuse for such a therapy: It helps."

That's the way Walter Kempner, M.D., a professor at Duke University Medical School, Durham, North Carolina, described his new therapeutic diet to a 1944 meeting of the North Carolina Medical Society. Consisting almost exclusively of rice and fruit, the radical diet was extremely low in salt, fat and protein, yet sufficient in essential nutrients because it was supplemented with vitamins.

CRITICAL MOMENTS

A respected researcher from Germany, Dr. Kempner had originally developed his unusual diet in 1939 as a short-term treatment for critically ill patients. In a pivotal event in 1942, he prescribed it for a 33-year-old North Carolina farm woman who had checked into the hospital with high blood pressure, failing eyesight, kidney disease and an enlarged heart. After a few days on the rice diet, the woman was sent home with personal orders from the doctor to stay on the diet for two more weeks and then to return for a checkup.

The woman didn't return for two *months,* apparently having misunderstood Dr. Kempner's German accent. Worried at first, he was then amazed to see that her blood pressure had dropped to a normal level and her eyesight had significantly improved. She adhered to the strict diet for another two months and two years later, still following a modified form of the diet, she reported feeling "young and strong."

But the medical community was critical, wanting him to test his diet in scientific experiments rather than prescribing it directly to his patients. The same year as his lecture to doctors in North Carolina, Dr. Kempner presented his work in Chicago to a gathering of the American Medical Association, including "before" and "after" X-rays and photographs of some of the 150 patients he had successfully treated. A close colleague indignantly told him afterward that a doctor in the audience had charged that Dr. Kempner's exhibits were forgeries.

"If the only way they can explain what I did is to call it a forgery, I must have done something," Dr. Kempner replied.

WILD FOR RICE

Turning his back on the criticism, Dr. Kempner instead attended to his patients, who descended upon Durham in droves. The hospital was so crowded that patients who were less critically ill boarded in hotels or private homes nearby.

Essentially unchanged in 50 years, the diet today is still being prescribed at the one remaining rice house. Patients stay on the diet without interruption until all health problems are under optimal control. Then selected foods that don't make them sick all over again can be added.

Physicians who support Dr. Kempner's approach credit the diet with dramatic turnarounds in serious cases of high blood pressure and heart disease, diabetes, liver and kidney disease, arthritis and obesity.

If you have heard of the diet at all, you probably think of it as the super-duper weight-loss regimen described a couple of years ago in a best-selling paperback by a formerly fat Kempner patient. One reason for its success as a diet, some point out, is that its sheer monotony cuts down on one's appetite.

The rice diet is actually a forerunner to the healthy-for-your-heart Pritikin Diet and other therapeutic meal plans, says Robert Rosati, M.D., a Duke University cardiologist who now prescribes the rice diet for patients with coronary artery disease.

"This diet is an extremely effective treatment. I've seen people who were too sick for bypass surgery get well on the diet. People come to the foundation blind from diabetes and go away able to see. Others have avoided kidney dialysis," he says.

"Somebody has to show people that there's a way they can take care of themselves to get healthy and to stay healthy. Dr. Kempner has done that," says Dr. Rosati.

INTENSIVE HEALING RECIPE:
RICE DIET

This salt-free rice dish is an example of the types of meals allowed to patients on the Rice Diet. The recipe appeared in the 1982 Bulletin of the Walter Kempner Foundation.

Rice, a staple of the world's diet, offers magnesium and a hefty amount of fiber.

PILAFF

2   cups uncooked rice
4   cups water
1   medium onion, chopped
1   clove garlic, chopped
½   cup apple juice
1   or 2 tsp. lemon juice

Place rice in a 1-quart saucepan (preferably aluminum without a nonstick coating) with a tight-fitting lid. Do not add oil or water. Cover and cook over medium-high heat, stirring frequently, until rice is uniformly golden brown. Reduce heat to low.

In a 2½-quart sauce-pan, bring water to a boil.

Remove lid from rice pan and add about one-third of the boiling water. When you see a burst of steam, cover immediately and keep covered until hissing stops. Add another one-third of the water, stir *once* and cover until water is absorbed, about 5 minutes. Then add remaining water, cover and let stand until it is absorbed.

Add onions, garlic, apple juice and lemon juice to rice and stir to combine. Turn off heat, cover pan and let stand until the hot rice has cooked the onions.

The pilaff may be served immediately or refrigerated and heated as needed in a colander over boiling water or in the microwave.

Variation: Along with the onions, garlic and juices, add a small amount of sherry or white wine in which some raisins have been simmered. Also, for some extra color and zest, add a few tomato slices before serving.

Yield: 4 servings

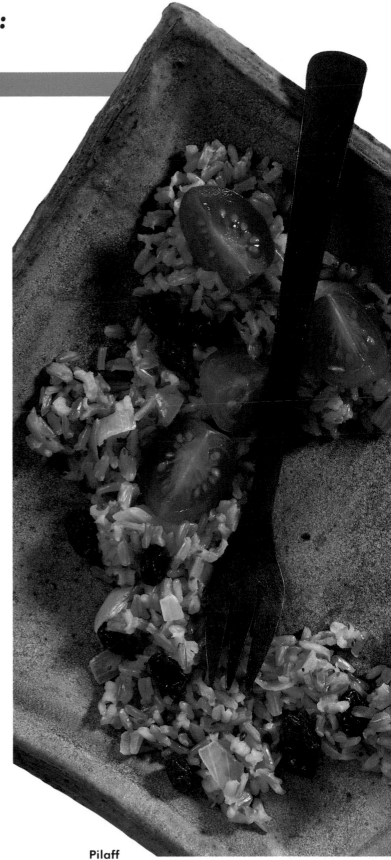

Pilaff

LACTOSE INTOLERANCE

If you are one of the 50 million adult Americans battling lactose intolerance—if you see milk as a pistol-toting warrior just waiting to shred your digestive system, leaving you with gas, bloating and diarrhea—then don't be surprised if yogurt, with flag flying, rides to your rescue, ready to wipe out those pesky symptoms.

At least that's the latest bulletin from researchers on the front line. Their studies indicate that if you are lactose intolerant—if your body is unable to digest the sugar in milk and many other dairy products—eating yogurt every day can increase your ability to consume dairy products without becoming a victim of uncomfortable symptoms.

MAKING YOGURT

If you are lactose intolerant and your body sings the blues every time you try to drink milk or have a milk product, you might want to consider making friends with yogurt. Yogurt is usually easily digestible by lactose-intolerant people, and new studies show that eating yogurt every day may completely eliminate or reduce the symptoms of lactose intolerance.

If you want the fun of making your own yogurt, here's a simple recipe.

First, heat fresh milk to just below boiling. A quart of milk (skim, whole, even half-and-half) will make a quart of yogurt. Next, allow the milk to cool until tepid. Then stir in 2 to 3 heaping tablespoons of plain, prepared yogurt with live cultures and beat until blended with milk. Then pour the mixture into a yogurt maker and let it incubate for four to six hours.

You don't have a yogurt maker? No problem. Just pour the mixture into a wide-mouthed Thermos. Or "hatch" it in a covered glass bowl in a warm place, such as an oven that has been preheated to 120°F and turned off. Do not disturb the culture while it is forming.

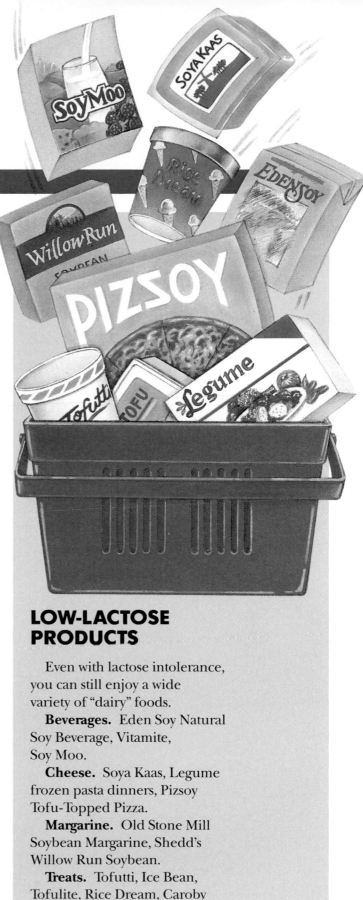

"Eating yogurt is a natural cure for lactose intolerance. At this time, it appears to be a novel and creative way of dealing with the problem," says Naresh Jain, M.D., a gastroenterologist from Our Lady of Mercy Medical Center in New York City.

RELIEF IN A WEEK

Dr. Jain and his team had five lactose-intolerant adults eat 6 ounces of unflavored yogurt twice a day for seven days. After just a week, two of them became completely lactose tolerant, and two others were dramatically relieved of their previous symptoms. The fifth person had a slight reduction in symptoms.

As for yogurt, feel free to indulge in flavored as well as unflavored types. But be wary of both frozen and "repasteurized" yogurt. Because of the extra processing involved in producing these products, the benefits to the lactose intolerant may be reduced, according to Dennis A. Savaiano, Ph.D., an associate professor in the Department of Food Science and Nutrition at the University of Minnesota at St. Paul.

The key to making yogurt work for you, according to Dr. Savaiano and other experts, is to select the type in which the cultures are live.

Why does yogurt give you a break when other dairy products don't? "Our studies suggest that yogurt comes with its own digestive enzyme," Dr. Savaiano says, "an enzyme that allows yogurt's lactose to be digested in the small intestine."

A KINDER COW

But, you say, you're not willing to eat yogurt twice a day, every day, for an indefinite time. What about treating yourself to treated milk products, which contain added lactase (the enzyme your body is missing)? Lactase-treated milk (such as Lactaid) has the same nutrient value as untreated milk and tastes about the same. Lactase also comes in capsule form. Pop a few of these before you eat any dairy food and—if you're not abnormally intolerant—you should note that after drinking your vanilla shake or eating your hot fudge sundae, all you feel is sinfully satisfied.

LOW-LACTOSE PRODUCTS

Even with lactose intolerance, you can still enjoy a wide variety of "dairy" foods.

Beverages. Eden Soy Natural Soy Beverage, Vitamite, Soy Moo.

Cheese. Soya Kaas, Legume frozen pasta dinners, Pizsoy Tofu-Topped Pizza.

Margarine. Old Stone Mill Soybean Margarine, Shedd's Willow Run Soybean.

Treats. Tofutti, Ice Bean, Tofulite, Rice Dream, Caroby Milkfree Bar.

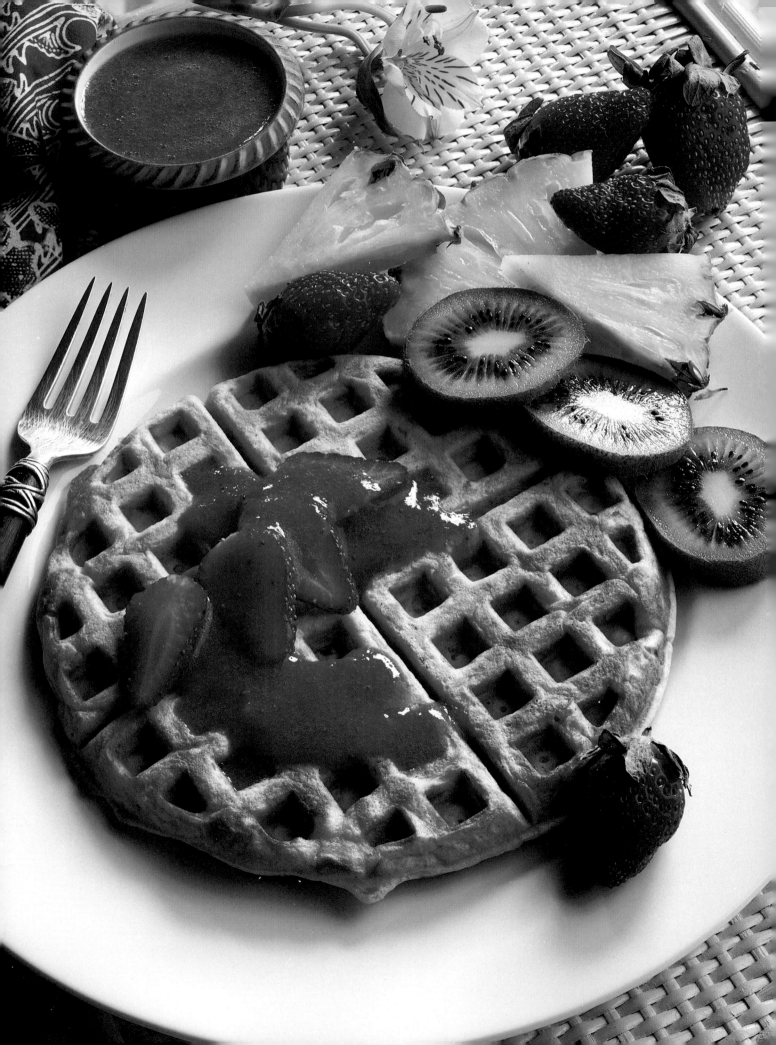

INTENSIVE HEALING RECIPES:
LACTOSE INTOLERANCE

Because of the restriction on the use of milk, people with lactose intolerance may worry about a calcium deficiency. But consider Apricot-Pecan Waffles with Strawberry Coulis, which offer nondairy calcium. Or imagine preparing Creamy Broccoli Soup without having to use any cream. It, too, is loaded with calcium.

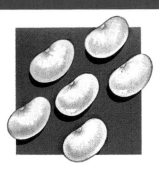

Even with lactose intolerance, there's no need to pass up our Creamy Broccoli Soup. The "cream" is actually pureed white beans—loaded with fiber.

APRICOT-PECAN WAFFLES WITH STRAWBERRY COULIS

Waffles
- ¾ cup unbleached flour
- ¾ cup whole wheat pastry flour
- 1½ tsp. baking powder
- ⅓ to ½ cup chopped pecans
- 1¼ cups apricot nectar
- 1½ Tbsp. safflower oil
- 2 eggs, lightly beaten, at room temperature
- 3 Tbsp. maple syrup

Coulis
- 1 cup fresh or partially thawed frozen strawberries
- ¼ cup apricot nectar
- 2 Tbsp. maple syrup

To make the waffles:
Preheat a waffle iron.

In a large bowl, sift together flours and baking powder. Stir in pecans.

In a medium-size bowl, whisk apricot nectar, oil, eggs and maple syrup. Then, using a large rubber spatula, add wet ingredients to dry ingredients, using as few strokes as possible.

When the waffle iron is hot, use a pastry brush to brush the grids with a bit of oil. Then pour in enough batter to cover two-thirds of the bottom grids. Bake according to manufacturer's directions but note that these waffles (because they don't contain milk) will take slightly less time than regular waffles. Start checking to see if they are done after 3 minutes. Continue brushing the grids with oil and baking waffles until batter is gone.

To make the coulis:
Place strawberries, apricot nectar and maple syrup in a food processor and process until smooth.

Serve waffles hot, with coulis drizzled over them.

Yield: 4 servings

CREAMY BROCCOLI SOUP

- 2 tsp. olive oil
- 1 medium onion, finely chopped
- 1 lb. broccoli, trimmed and chopped
- 1 bay leaf
- 3 allspice berries, crushed
- 1 cup cooked white beans
- 2 cups stock
  Chopped tomato or sweet red or yellow pepper strips, for garnish

Heat oil in a large stockpot. Add onions and sauté until quite brown, about 15 minutes. Add broccoli, bay leaf, allspice, beans and stock and bring to a boil.

Reduce heat to simmer, cover loosely and simmer until broccoli is tender, about 20 minutes.

Let soup cool slightly and remove bay leaf.

Place soup in a food processor or blender and process until very smooth. (If necessary, process in two batches.) Serve hot, garnished with tomatoes or peppers.

Yield: 4 servings

NACHOS

- 4 corn tortillas
- ½ cup refried beans
- 1 Tbsp. plus 1 tsp. salsa
- ½ cup crumbled mild goat cheese or grated soy cheese (not tofu)

Preheat the oven to 400°F.

Set tortillas directly on a middle oven rack and bake until crisp but not brown, about 5 minutes.

Use an icing spatula to spread refried beans on tortillas. Then spread on salsa and last, the cheese.

Then carefully cut tortillas into quarters with kitchen scissors. Set quarters on a slotted broiler rack and bake until cheese has softened or melted, about 3 minutes. Serve warm with extra salsa on the side.

Yield: 4 servings

Apricot-Pecan Waffles with Strawberry Coulis

THE MASTER HEALING DIET

Optimal health. You want it, you deserve it and you're willing to go to great lengths to get it. Knowing that diet makes a difference, you're all revved up to do a number on your nutrition, whether it's wolfing down wheat germ or cutting out cookies—whatever it takes.

A bit of advice: Slow down, because it really doesn't take that much. Just eat your vegetables and fresh fruits, plus a selection of grains, seafood and poultry, low-fat dairy products and cholesterol-free oils—all foods proven to be powerful health-builders as well as agents in healing.

As an aid in your design of a dynamite diet, we've compiled this comprehensive chart of 50 "super foods." Every one of them has undergone scientific scrutiny and been found to be linked to the prevention or treatment of a number of disorders, from cancer to overweight.

As part of a healing lunch, for instance, munch a bunch of broccoli, which scores in all seven of our categories. Studies have suggested that eating a diet

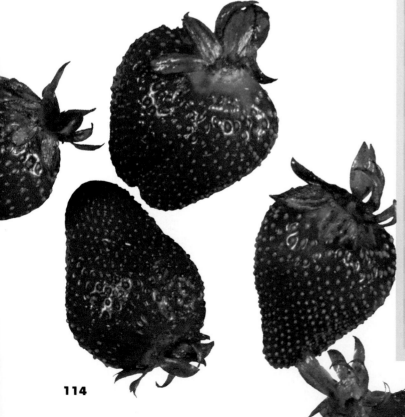

FIFTY SUPERFOODS THAT HEAL

	CANCER	
ALMONDS, UNSALTED		
APPLES	⊂ɪɪɪ	
APRICOTS	⊂ɪɪɪ	
ASPARAGUS	⊂ɪɪɪ	
AVOCADOS		
BANANAS	⊂ɪɪɪ	
BARLEY	⊂ɪɪɪ	
BROCCOLI	⊂ɪɪɪ	
BROWN RICE	⊂ɪɪɪ	
CABBAGE	⊂ɪɪɪ	
CANTALOUPE	⊂ɪɪɪ	
CARROTS	⊂ɪɪɪ	
CAULIFLOWER	⊂ɪɪɪ	
CELERY	⊂ɪɪɪ	
CORN	⊂ɪɪɪ	
EGGPLANT	⊂ɪɪɪ	
GRAPEFRUIT	⊂ɪɪɪ	
GREEN PEAS	⊂ɪɪɪ	
GREEN PEPPERS	⊂ɪɪɪ	
HONEYDEW	⊂ɪɪɪ	
KALE	⊂ɪɪɪ	
LENTILS		
MACKEREL		
NECTARINES	⊂ɪɪɪ	
OAT BRAN	⊂ɪɪɪ	

HIGH BLOOD PRESSURE	STROKE	CHOLESTEROL	HEART DISEASE	OSTEO-POROSIS	OVERWEIGHT
✓	✓		✓	✓	
✓	✓		✓		✓
✓	✓		✓		✓
✓	✓		✓		✓
✓	✓	✓			
✓	✓	✓	✓		✓
✓		✓			
✓	✓	✓	✓	✓	✓
✓	✓	✓	✓		✓
✓	✓	✓	✓		✓
✓	✓		✓		✓
	✓	✓	✓		✓
✓					✓
	✓				✓
	✓		✓		✓
✓					✓
✓	✓		✓		✓
✓	✓		✓		✓
	✓		✓		✓
✓			✓		✓
	✓		✓	✓	✓
	✓	✓	✓		✓
✓	✓	✓	✓	✓	
✓	✓		✓		✓
		✓			✓

(continued)

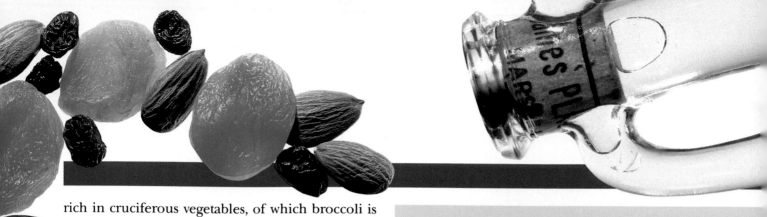

rich in cruciferous vegetables, of which broccoli is one, may decrease *cancer* risks; broccoli is also packed with beta-carotene and vitamin C, two powerful cancer fighters. Broccoli is rich in the mineral potassium, related to a lowered incidence of *hypertension* and *stroke*. Its high fiber also helps lower your *cholesterol* level, which, along with the vegetable's low-salt and low-fat content, lowers your chances of *heart disease*. Broccoli is a great source of bone-building calcium, which can reduce your chances of developing *osteoporosis*. Finally, broccoli gives *overweight* the double whammy: not only is it very low in calories but its high fiber helps fill you up.

Some foods high on our health scale may be unfamiliar to you. We've all nibbled corn, but what about kale? (Hint: It's green and leafy like lettuce.) Everybody has feasted on turkey, but tofu? (It's a form of soybeans.) Try something you've never tasted before. Experiment with new recipes and add special touches of your own.

Most importantly, remember that a lifetime habit of healthy eating begins with meals that you truly enjoy. *Bon appetit!*

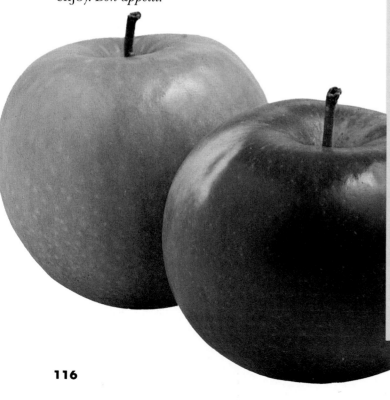

FIFTY SUPERFOODS—Continued

	CANCER	
OLIVE OIL		
ONIONS	⬛	
ORANGES	⬛	
PEACHES	⬛	
PEANUTS, UNSALTED		
POTATOES	⬛	
PRUNES		
RAISINS	⬛	
SAFFLOWER OIL		
SALMON	⬛	
SARDINES	⬛	
SKIM MILK	⬛	
SPINACH	⬛	
STRAWBERRIES	⬛	
SUNFLOWER SEEDS	⬛	
SWEET POTATOES	⬛	
SWISS CHARD	⬛	
TOFU	⬛	
TOMATOES	⬛	
TUNA		
TURKEY, WHITE MEAT, NO SKIN		
WATERMELON	⬛	
WHOLE GRAIN CEREAL	⬛	
WINTER SQUASH	⬛	
YOGURT, LOW-FAT	⬛	

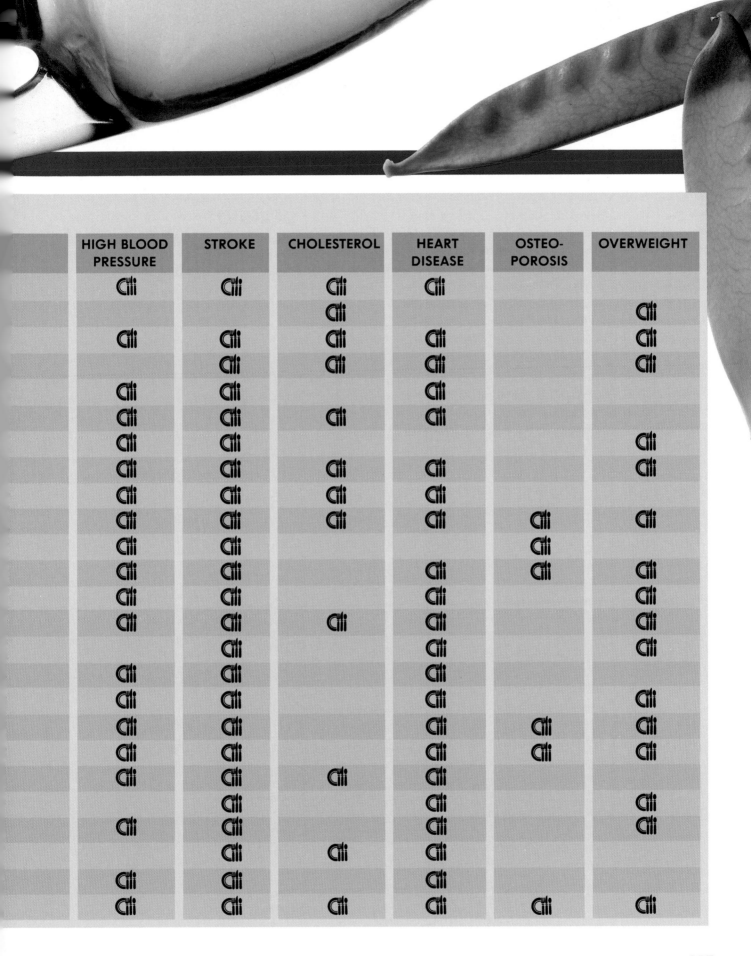

MEDICAL CARE AND YOUR HEALING DIET

Mmmmm! You're cooking up something really special. You're whipping up a tasty treat certain to satisfy your *healthiest* appetite—the appetite for life, for energy and strength and wellness day after day. Naturally, you use only the finest ingredients: whole grains, fresh fruits and vegetables, low-fat dairy products. But remember to add one very important ingredient to your new recipe for health: your doctor.

Many of us see a physician on a regular basis, entrusting him or her to monitor our health. Enlist his help in making major dietary changes, too, advises Arlene Caggiula, Ph.D., associate professor of nutrition and epidemiology at the University of Pittsburgh School of Public Health.

PARTNERS IN HEALTH

Who is responsible for your health? You are, ultimately. But this responsibility includes forging a partnership with a doctor who has the kind of expertise you need to make dietary changes wisely and safely. The doctors we interviewed explain why.

Diagnosis. Before you make any kind of dietary change to prevent or treat a disease, you need to see a doctor to determine whether you're really a candidate for the disease. "Don't go on a diet to try to prevent diabetes, for example, if you show no symptoms or have no family history of the disease," says Hans Fisher, Ph.D., chairman of the Department of Nutrition at Rutgers University.

If you strongly suspect you really might have a problem, you should find out how bad it is. "If you learn it's a real problem, you're going to be better motivated to do something about it," says Paul D. Thompson, M.D., a cardiologist and associate professor of medicine at Brown University.

Objectivity. "Most people don't really know what their eating habit problems are," says Dr. Caggiula, who helps patients reduce their high blood pressure through a nutritional program developed especially for that purpose. Even if you know you need to cut back on certain foods, "few people know much about the sodium or fat or cholesterol content of specific foods, let alone the relative importance of each of these substances in their diet." A nutritionally aware physician can help you determine where you need to make changes and how to most effectively do so.

Medical complications. Are you taking medi-

WHEN *NOT* TO SEE YOUR DOCTOR

Our expert agrees: Go ahead and practice medicine on your own without the aid of a physician—as long as it's of the *preventive* sort. You can be your own best doctor when it comes to changing "high-risk" health habits linked to heart disease and a number of other disorders.

"The American Heart Association directly advertises its 'prudent diet' to individuals," says Joseph Stokes, M.D. "It doesn't depend on health professionals to get that important message across. Just be sure to get your regular medical checkups. Then you need only check with your doctor if you encounter problems or have questions."

Many recommendations published by national medical panels—eat less fat or eat more fiber, for example—often don't require physician consultation. Nevertheless, it's still a good idea to check with your doctor. Then go ahead and follow the diet, checking back in two weeks to see if it's making a difference.

"When it comes to making lifestyle changes—losing weight, stopping smoking, exercising—people not only have to want to do these things for themselves but must feel they have the personal power to do them, " says Steven Jonas, M.D. "These are the people who have the most success."

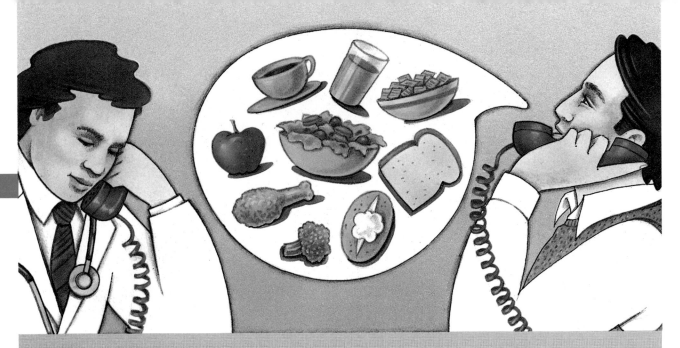

DIAL-A-DOC

Marvin Mordkoff, M.D., doesn't make house calls—he makes phone calls. As part of a special "Phone-In Program," hundreds of his patients call every week to report on the status of their weight, diet and other health factors. While they're on the line, they can get free nutritional and medical advice.

"Any physician can make a diagnosis," he says. "But it's compliance that counts. The best results are achieved with ongoing communication." Communication—the essence of medical care.

cine for a disease? Your medications could interact with changes in your diet. Patients taking certain drugs prescribed for high blood pressure, for instance, should not eat foods that increase their levels of the mineral potassium, says Dr. Caggiula.

Some people also believe that following a diet for certain diseases can enable them to go off medications completely, says Dr. Fisher. Don't do it, he says. See your doctor first.

HOW TO TALK TO YOUR DOCTOR

First things first: "Make sure your doctor is an expert in the nutrition-related aspects of disease," says Dr. Fisher. Unfortunately, not all doctors are.

If your current doctor isn't well-versed in nutrition, "ask him to refer you to a registered nutritionist," says Steven Jonas, M.D., a professor of preventive medicine at the State University of New York, Stony Brook. "The next best thing is to make an appointment with a nutritionist at your local hospital." (For more information, see the entry on nutritionists, beginning on page 130.)

But give your present doctor a chance. "It's sometimes difficult to tell your doctor what you want, but you have to do it," says Dr. Jonas.

"Ask questions. Be assertive," says Joseph Stokes, M.D., professor of medicine at Boston University Medical Center. "I've seen situations where patients are pushing their doctor, asking questions he or she finds difficult to answer. That's very motivating. The doctor will go out and find the answers. As a result, patients will get better and better advice."

KEYS TO SUCCESS

"You need a lot of inner motivation to follow any diet," says Dr. Jonas. "One of the most important roles a doctor plays is helping you develop that motivation." Dr. Jonas offers these other helpful hints.

Set reasonable goals. Determine what you're trying to accomplish and, with your doctor, set goals. These will increase your likelihood of success.

Get things straight. Make sure you understand your doctor's advice. For example, if he uses the words "glycogen" and "glucose," ask him to use the more common term: sugar. Ask him, too, for any written materials he might have on the subject.

Check back. A good doctor cares enough to set up a regular schedule of revisits to check on your progress. Demonstrate that *you* care, too. Show up for follow-up appointments even if you're positive everything is fine.

NATURAL FOOD ADVOCATES

These are "fringe" health gurus of the 20th century. They believed in natural foods, exercise and, often, things like enemas. They didn't believe in doctors. Millions of Americans believed in *them*.

"Charlatans!" says Stanley Gershoff, Ph.D., dean of the Tufts University School of Nutrition, pointing to their contention that any diet but their own leads to "malnutrition." "It's patently absurd that we're all malnourished. Just look around!"

On the other hand, some of their ideas have moved from fringe to mainstream: the value of fiber, of fresh fruits and vegetables, of exercise.

One thing is for certain: Most of these people were their own best advertisement. Through their own methods—however extreme—they lived, and continue to live, extraordinary lives.

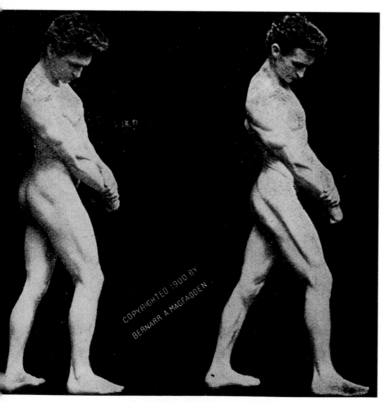

Bernarr Macfadden lost 15 pounds (right) after seven days without food. But he still found the strength to hoist a 100-pound dumbbell over his head.

BERNARR MACFADDEN

Bernarr Macfadden was the most colorful of them all. When he died in 1955 at age 87, the *New York Times* called him a "health faddist, publishing titan. political aspirant, daredevil parachutist, penny-a-meal restaurateur . . . [and] a crusader with followers in the millions."

His life was an offbeat Horatio Alger tale come true. He was born in 1868 in a two-room Missouri cabin. Orphaned by age ten, he was a frail child, but exercised to improve himself. He came to New York as a young man, with $50 in his pocket. There he began teaching exercise classes—and the rest is, indeed, history.

Macfadden's publications reached millions of readers. *Physical Culture* magazine operated for 50 years, preaching vegetarianism and exercise and featuring inspiring displays of robust flesh. He also pioneered titillating formats with publications like *True Story, The Romance,* and the *New York Evening Graphic,* a news tabloid that put some of the roar into the twenties: It was nicknamed the "porno-Graphic."

Macfadden practiced the physical culture he preached. Even as a senior citizen, he walked several miles a day, played tennis and, of course, leapt from airplanes. On his 83rd birthday he made a 2,500-foot parachute jump into the Hudson River in New York; a year later, he pulled a similar stunt over Paris.

He had political aspirations—he sought to be mayor and governor of New York—but perhaps the scandal surrounding his three marriages prevented those dreams from coming true. At 84, he moved from New York City to nearby Jersey City to escape high alimony payments. He had lost most of his millions by then.

His reluctance to pay alimony notwithstanding, Macfadden's philanthropy was celebrated. He donated millions of dollars to set up schools, foundations and associations to promote physical culture. During the depression, his New York restaurants offered meals to the masses for the right price: a penny.

PAUL BRAGG

In 1973, a reporter for Knight Newspapers met fitness guru Paul Bragg. She was impressed. "Seen on the street from a distance of 6 feet or so, he might be taken for 55," she wrote. "A bit closer, and the casual observer could decide he's 50."

Not bad: Bragg was 92 at the time. Like his mentor Bernarr Macfadden, Paul Bragg was a superstar. Millions attended his "Bragg Crusades," listened to his radio and TV programs and bought his books. His clients included the most famous names of their day: Gloria Swanson, Conrad Hilton and Sugar Ray Robinson, plus one sickly, pimply, suicidal teenager, who under his tutelage metamorphosed into Jack La Lanne.

Bragg was also a marketing pioneer and is credited with establishing the first health food store and with commercializing a wide variety of health products, like vitamins, tomato juice, seven-grain cereals and health cosmetics.

But most of all, there was his energy—the man was bursting with it, judging from the corny photographs that adorn many of his 40 books. There's Bragg waterskiing, the firm muscles of his massive body impressively displayed by his brief bikini; Bragg roller skating, in very short shorts; Bragg frolicking, nearly nude, in the snow. Usually, his head is thrown back, roaring with delight at his vibrant good health.

He lived by his adage, "To rest is to rust." At 88, he was the nation's 19th-ranked senior tennis player. His daily regimen at that age included a two-mile run, a headstand ("Standing on your head adds years to your face!") and a cold shower. Half his diet was raw fruits and vegetables, and he also ate some meats, fish and natural cheeses. He took vitamins, fasted regularly and practiced breathing exercises picked up from an Indian holy man. He crusaded for sunshine and good posture and against white sugar, white flour, salt, pesticides, chemical additives, coffee, alcohol and tobacco.

Like many others of his ilk, Bragg's interest in health grew out of early illness. Born in Virginia, he

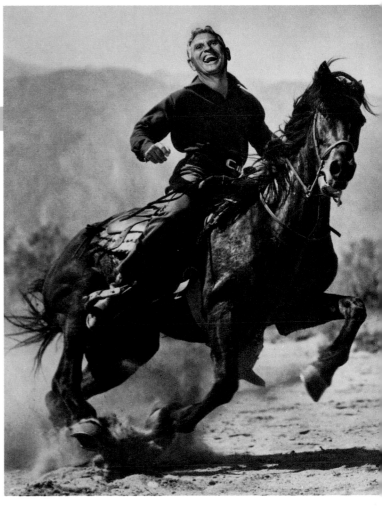

Exuding the gusto of good health, Paul Bragg rides his favorite bronco, Dynamite, at his western ranch. The high-held head was a Bragg trademark. So was the robust image.

contracted tuberculosis at 16 and was sent to Switzerland for a cure. There he became interested in natural therapies. He studied at Oxford University and earned a Ph.D. in biochemistry. He also studied naturopathy and homeopathic medicine. In 1903, he became Bernarr Macfadden's right-hand man at *Physical Culture* magazine. He moved to California in 1918.

Bragg called himself a "life extension specialist" and would say that he expected to live past 120. He came closer than most. But a few months after a swimming accident that damaged his lungs, he succumbed to a heart attack at age 95.

At Bragg's funeral, a message from Jack La Lanne was read: "Paul Bragg saved my life . . . . His dedicated gifts of love and inspiration and the hope he has given countless thousands shall never be forgotten. He was, and is still, my lifeline."

ARNOLD EHRET

"Lesson 1. Every disease, no matter what name it is known by Medical Science, is Constipation, a clogging up of the entire pipe system of the human body."

So began Arnold Ehret's 1922 classic, *Mucusless Diet Healing System*. Never mind World War I: In the early part of the century, Ehret's approach split many Europeans and Americans into battling camps of Ehretists and non-Ehretists.

He started out as an art professor from Baden, Germany, who suffered from kidney trouble and "consumptive tendencies." At 31, he commenced a worldwide search for cures. Finally, in Algiers, he found that a fruit diet combined with fasting brought him the energy and health he craved.

Years later, he would fondly recall the moment when his "constipation" was finally relieved: "After a two years' cure . . . by fasting and strict living on a mucusless diet, I ate 2 pounds of the sweetest grapes and drank half a gallon of fresh, sweet grape juice. . . . Almost immediately I felt as though I were going to die! A terrible sensation overcame me, palpitation of the heart, extreme dizziness . . . . After ten minutes the great event occurred—diarrhea and vomiting of grape juice—and then the greatest event of all . . . . I felt so wonderfully well and strong that I at once performed knee-bending and arm-stretching exercises 326 times consecutively. All obstructions had been removed!"

Ehret went on to electrify Europe with his feats of physical endurance, his lengthy public fasts—of a month or more—his articles and the cures he supervised. He immigrated to the United States just before World War I.

Ehret's theory was that certain foods caused "mucus" (decayed wastes) to accumulate in the body, creating disease. The cure involved eating fibrous foods: cooked and raw fruits and nonstarchy vegetables, and some whole grains. Forbidden foods included meats, eggs, milk, white flour, legumes and rice. Periodic fasting would speed the cleansing process.

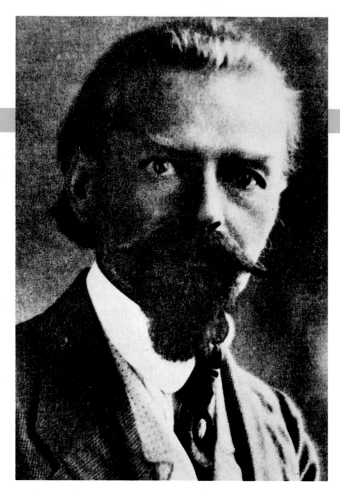

"My system is not a cure, it is a housecleaning," claimed Arnold Ehret, the art professor who became a self-styled authority on the lower bowel.

Ehret also displayed a discomforting interest in "eugenics," breeding a superior race of men through abstinence. "Why did the birth of boy babies increase during the European war?" he asked. "Restriction in diet and restriction in sexual intercourse, that is all! The cleaner the body of both parents, the less frequent the intercourse, the smaller the quantity of food, the greater the love vibrations become, and with these conditions the better the chance for a genius and that is always a boy."

Ehret also believed in enemas and exercise, but he wasn't a complete killjoy: His "airbath" prescription sounds like fun. "A few minutes each day spent before an open window upon arising and just before retiring, when all clothes are removed, massaging the body—helps the skin to retain its natural functioning qualities."

Ehret died at 56, after a fall on an oil-soaked driveway in Los Angeles.

PAAVO AIROLA

Your local health food store, or even your public library, probably stocks some of the books of Paavo Airola. *Are You Confused?*, *How to Get Well*, *Health Secrets from Europe*, and other titles have sold upwards of five *million* copies.

If you flip through one of those books—even those written nearly 20 years ago—the contemporary tone may surprise you. "It is somewhat ironic that after decades of study, the cornerstones of Airola's teachings turned out to be surprisingly simple," concluded *Vegetarian Times* magazine in a 1983 eulogy of their columnist. "Eat a well-balanced, grain-centered vegetarian diet, get sufficient exercise and have a healthy, positive mental attitude."

An international perspective brought Airola to those simple principles. Born in Europe in 1918, he studied art as a young man. A World War II injury spurred his interest in health, and he went on to receive a Ph.D. in biochemistry and a degree in naturopathy. Airola then spent years studying the diets of native cultures around the world.

From these studies, he evolved a system that he called "biological medicine." His premise was that most diseases are caused by physical and mental stresses, which can include "constant overeating, overindulgence in proteins . . . nutritional deficiencies, sluggish metabolism and consequent retention of toxic metabolic wastes, exogenous poisons from polluted food, water, air and environment, toxic drugs, tobacco and alcohol, lack of sufficient exercise . . . severe emotional and physical stresses, etc. . . . Bacteria is more often than not the *result* of disease, not its *cause*."

A typical Airola prescription to overcome health problems—ranging from acne and alcoholism to varicose veins and warts—might include a juice fast, vitamins, kelp, brewer's yeast, lecithin, herbs, massage and exercise. A vegetarian diet, he felt, is essential. And, long before conventional medicine confirmed the "relaxation response," he preached peace of mind.

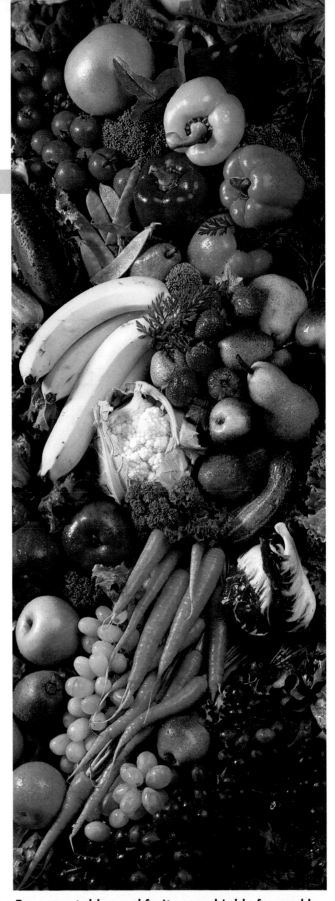

Raw vegetables and fruits were highly favored by naturopath Paavo Airola. He maintained that cooking destroyed vital enzymes in food and interfered with digestion.

123

HERBERT M. SHELTON

The baby had pneumonia, and no less than five physicians agreed that the child was doomed. The desperate mother called a professional hygienist. His advice went like this:

"Go to the table at the bedside of your baby and sweep all the boxes and bottles of drugs that are there into the wastebasket. Next, open the window and let some fresh air into the room . . . . Give the baby as much water as it wants, but no food and no more drugs."

The child recovered and grew to "splendid young womanhood," related Herbert Shelton in *Fasting Can Save Your Life*. This was one of many stories intended to demonstrate the power of Natural Hygiene, a healing system that involved natural foods, fasting and avoidance of physicians.

Natural Hygiene was invented in the 19th century by crusaders like Sylvester Graham, pioneer of vegetarianism and whole grains. There was much to commend—like advocacy of natural foods and sanitation—and to condemn—like blood leeching

FOR BETTER OR WORSE

Natural Hygienists believe you should eat only certain fruits, vegetables, grains, nuts and seeds—even these foods have to be properly "combined" at each meal to make their way healthfully through the digestive tract.

BAD COMBINATIONS	GOOD COMBINATIONS
Fruits and seeds	Fruits together
Fruits and nuts	Vegetables together
Grains and seeds	Vegetables and nuts
Grains and nuts	Vegetables and seeds
Vegetables and fruits	Vegetables and grains
Grains and fruits	Melons alone

and withholding food from the sick. By the start of the 20th century, the movement was all but dead.

Shelton, a sharecropper's son who was born in Wylie, Texas, in 1895, discovered the writings of the natural hygienists when he was 16. He went on to earn degrees in chiropractic and naturopathy but grew to distrust their unpredictable "cures."

So he dug out the principles of Natural Hygiene, stripped away some of the hocus-pocus (like the leeches), and put them into practice.

He succeeded. Dr. Shelton's Health School was founded in San Antonio, Texas, in 1928, and more than 40,000 people were treated there before it closed in 1981. His magazine, *Dr. Shelton's Hygienic Review*, launched in 1939, was published through 1980. He also wrote more than 40 books.

Exercise, fresh air and moderation were all important to Natural Hygiene, but for Shelton, fasting was the key component. He supervised thousands of fasts and advised careful fasting for everything from asthma to infertility.

"Fasting in itself has no force," he wrote, "but rather it enables the body's organs and recuperative forces to turn their full energies on the problem to be corrected."

Mahatma Gandhi was reportedly interested in Shelton's work and invited him to visit India, but the outbreak of World War II interceded.

Shelton was a philosopher, a man of principle and a pacifist. He opposed America's entry into the war, and he gave up an opportunity to have his own radio program because he refused to endorse the would-be sponsor's laxative.

Shelton died in 1985 at age 89. But his work lives on. The American Natural Hygiene Society, of which he was cofounder, is thriving in Tampa, Florida. (Although, according to Executive Director James M. Lennon, many of Shelton's more extreme views—like avoidance of physicians—have been modified.) In fact, the movement is enjoying unprecedented popularity because of Harvey and Marilyn Diamond's best-selling book *Fit for Life*. Their program adapts Shelton's theories on food combining.

NORMAN W. WALKER

Norman Walker was the juice man. He popularized fresh fruit and vegetable juices as health drinks in the United States. You thought juice bars were a recent phenomenon? Some *70* years ago, he had trendy Californians bellying up to a bar to sip his freshly squeezed formulations.

Walker was born in England before the turn of the century. As an ambitious young businessman, he suffered a breakdown and retreated to a peasant home in the French countryside. "One morning I happened to go into the kitchen while the old lady was peeling carrots for lunch," Walker recalled. "Watching her, I noticed how moist these carrots were when peeled. . . .

"That afternoon I asked her permission to pick a few carrots and to peel them. And could I use her feed grinder?" And that, says Walker, is how "I obtained my first introduction to a cupful of beautiful carrot juice!"

Walker recovered, and around 1910 he brought his enthusiasm for juices to Long Beach, California, where he teamed up with a medical doctor. Together they developed dozens of fresh juice formulas for specific medical conditions. (He recommended those

"The *life* in your food is what counts," claimed Norman Walker. And for him, fresh, raw vegetable juice was the perfect place to find it in abundance.

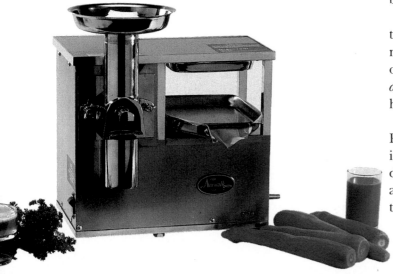

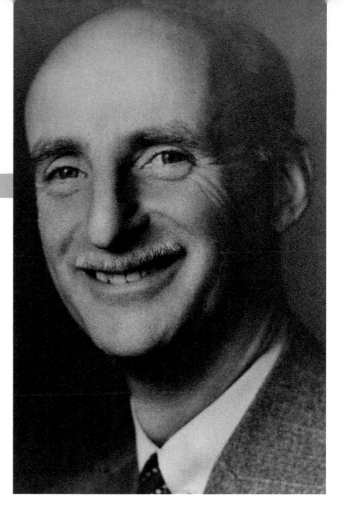

In 1934, Norman Walker began marketing a fresh fruit and vegetable juicer of his own invention. It's called the Norwalk Juicer, and it's still on the market today.

along with enemas and a vegetarian diet.) They opened a juice bar and even a juice delivery service. From 1910 to 1930, he was something of a national celebrity.

Colon status was also a major concern. "*Good morning!* How is your colon this morning? This is an excellent question for you to ask yourself, particularly when you wake up feeling logy, heavy, dull, listless and negative," Walker advised in one of his books.

Walker was also famous for one thing he wouldn't talk about: his age. "I am in complete possession of my faculties and I am alive, alert, energetic and full of enthusiasm," he wrote in 1972. "How old am I? *I am ageless!*" Followers say he was well over 100 when he died in 1985.

Walker's publisher, Don Woodside of Norwalk Press in Phoenix, Arizona, says Walker's books sell in six figures each year—and sales are rising. "Today, doctors say that if you want to avoid cancer, eat fruits and vegetables. He was saying that in 1910. That's the reason for our growth."

VIKTORAS KULVINSKAS

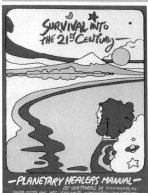

1968: an era of up-heaval. Viktoras Kul-vinskas, a 29-year-old computer researcher at the Massachusetts Insti-tute of Technology, is abusing alcohol, cigarettes and drugs. He has kidney problems, arthritis and graying hair. So he "retires."

He quits his job and moves into nutritionist Ann Wigmore's school. His health is transformed. He stays for seven years, help-ing Wigmore and researching other so-called New Age disciplines—numerology, iridology, color heal-ing. In 1975, he publishes *Survival into the 21st Century,* a dense catalog of advice on all these subjects and more. The message: The economic/environmental apocalypse is coming; prepare yourself. The book becomes a classic, selling more than 250,000 copies.

The late 1980s: an era of prosperity. Looking back on *Survival,* Kulvinskas comments that he was something of an "evangelistic fearmonger." Now he says, "Cataclysms can be avoided by consciousness changes."

His own consciousness has changed considerably. For one thing, his hair is shorter. (In *Survival* he had warned, "Haircuts can be dangerous to your health.") Kulvinskas lives and teaches in the "All-Life Sanctuary," his apartment in Manhattan's Chinatown. He offers low-key nutritional and spiritual counseling and promotes dietary supplements, like Super Blue-Green algae and digestive enzymes. Actor/activist Dick Gregory is his close friend and business partner, and Kulvinskas is co-creator of Gregory's Bahamian Diet powder, with millions of dollars in sales, and Nutritional Correction Connection, intended to help people overcome tobacco, drug, coffee and alcohol habits.

At 48, Kulvinskas is an extremely thin, intense but gentle man, who effortlessly twists himself into a

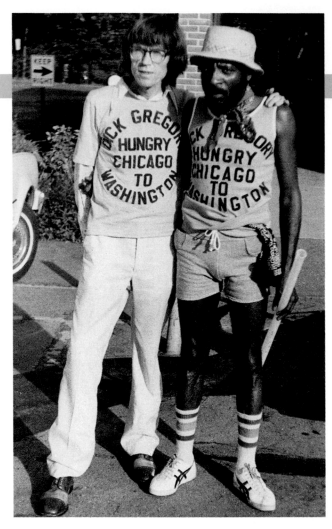

To demonstrate that a healthy body is a fit body, Viktoras Kulvinskas (left) joined friend Dick Gregory's 900-mile run to the nation's capital. The daily fare? Fruit juice.

tight yoga knot to demonstrate his complete recov-ery from arthritis. He agrees with his former mentor Ann Wigmore that disease arises out of malnutrition—from eating the wrong foods—and toxemia—caused by chemicals in food and the environment. But to Wigmore's Living Foods regimen, he adds a few cooked foods, plus vitamin, mineral and enzyme supplements, which are against Wigmore's teachings.

Kulvinskas is planning to move to the rural South to set up an institute to study life extension. "I see extending life span indefinitely as a possibility, up to two or three hundred years as a certainty," he says. One of the half-dozen books he is writing is called *From Longevity to Immortality.* "It will be a classic," he predicts.

ANN WIGMORE

Dozens of people live, study or eat there, but there are no stoves or refrigerators in the stately Boston mansion that houses the Ann Wigmore Foundation. Instead, there are simple wooden racks designed to hold trays of wheatgrass, sunflower sprouts and buckwheat sprouts.

On the outside, a mansion; on the inside, an organic farm, growing the "live foods" that Ann Wigmore says create health. "Dr. Ann," as devotees call her, is the woman who sparked the wheatgrass juice fad.

Her singular approach to nutrition came out of a rural Lithuanian childhood. She was born in 1909. Her grandmother was the village healer, whose "medicines" included crushed grasses. Wigmore came to the United States penniless and nearly lost her legs to gangrene after an accident. But she refused amputation. Instead, she ate wild grasses and recovered. Years later, she began studying grasses and hit upon wheatgrass as particularly high in chlorophyll, vitamins, minerals and enzymes.

Wigmore's diet prohibits cooking, which, she says, kills food's natural enzymes. Those enzymes, she maintains, are needed to digest food properly; improper digestion leads to malnutrition and disease. So do chemicals in food. Her program allows organically grown vegetables, fruits, grains, seeds, beans and nuts. But they must be eaten raw, grated, sprouted, blended, soaked, fermented, dehydrated —never, *ever* cooked.

A SPROUTING SAMPLER

For Ann Wigmore's students, sprouted seeds, beans and grains are staples. Here's a guide to some foods you "farm" in a jar.

VARIETY	SOAKING TIME (HRS.)	DRY MEASURE	LENGTH AT HARVEST (IN.)	SPROUTING TIME (DAYS)	SPROUTING TIPS	NUTRIENTS	SUGGESTED USES
ADZUKI	12	1 cup	½–1	3–5	Easy sprouter; try short and long	Protein, iron and calcium	Salads, oriental dishes, sandwiches, casseroles
ALFALFA	4–6	3 Tbsp.	1–1½	4–5	Place in light to develop chlorophyll 1–2 days before harvest	Protein, vitamins A, B, C, D, E, K and minerals	Salads, sandwiches, soups
CHICK-PEA	12	1 cup	½	2–3	Mix with lentils and wheat, or use alone	Protein and minerals	Dips, spreads, salads, casseroles
LENTIL	12	½ cup	¼–¾	3–5	Earthy flavor; try short and long; versatile	Protein, B vitamins and minerals	Spreads, salads, casseroles, soups
MUNG BEAN	12	½ cup	½–1½	3–5	Grow in dark; when rinsing, soak in cold water for 1 min.	Protein, vitamins A, B, C and minerals	Salads, oriental dishes, sandwiches

NOTE: Rinse and drain thoroughly twice a day for 3–5 days.

NUTRITIONAL BALANCE
AND YOUR HEALING DIET

"**A**ll right, class, it's time to name the four basic food groups. . . . "

If you learned anything about nutrition in grade school, it was the importance of a balanced diet. This, it was taught, was achieved by squeezing some grain, meat, dairy and fruit or vegetable into each day's meals.

Well, a lot has changed since the U.S. Department of Agriculture (USDA) first suggested the Basic Four. After all, when eggs were a dime a dozen, who ever heard of cholesterol?

Today, current guidelines divide food into six groups. The new system, says Anne Shaw, Ph.D., a nutritionist with the USDA, takes into account what modern science has learned, not only about cholesterol but also about sodium, sweeteners, fat and certain vitamins and minerals.

For all the changes, the basic premise has remained the same: "Choosing from a variety of foods helps protect you against nutritional deficiencies," says Dr. Shaw. "No one food can do that."

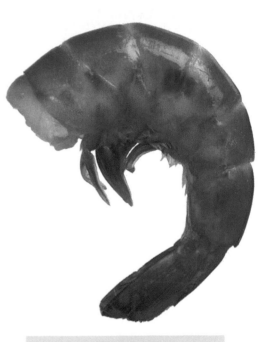

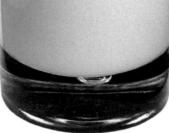

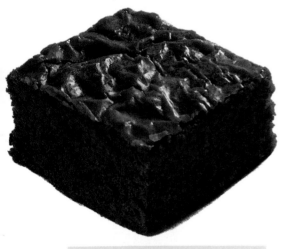

FOOD GROUP 3
Fish, poultry, meat and eggs are good sources of protein, niacin, zinc, and vitamins B_6 and B_{12}. The first three also contribute the most absorbable form of iron. *Two or three daily servings* (5 to 7 ounces total) are recommended. The best selections are the lowest in fat—choose baked fish, broiled chicken or roast turkey over greasy sausages, fat-laden frankfurters or luncheon meats. For vegetarians, appropriate substitutes are dried beans, peas, nuts and seeds. Remember, though, that vitamin B_{12} is found only in animal products. The same is true of cholesterol.

FOOD GROUP 2
Dairy products are good sources of protein, calcium, riboflavin, vitamin B_{12}, magnesium, vitamin A and thiamine. *Two daily servings* are recommended. Whether you choose milk, yogurt or cheese, always try to pick those lowest in fat. The best choices: nonfat yogurt, skim milk and buttermilk.

FOOD GROUP 1
Fats, sweets, and alcoholic beverages provide mainly calories. These foods should be consumed *in moderation* only.

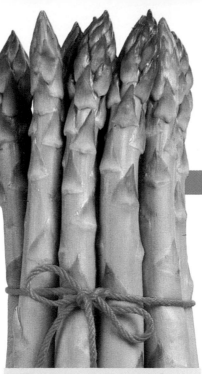

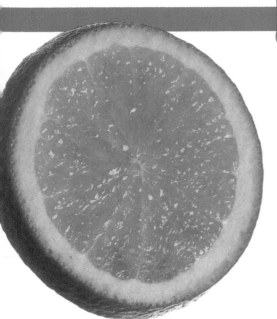

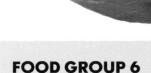

FOOD GROUP 4

Fruits contain varying amounts of many nutrients. Whole raw fruits, particularly those with edible skin, are good sources of fiber. Eat *two to four daily servings*. A serving might be an average-size whole fruit, a melon wedge, 6 ounces of fruit juice, ½ cup of berries or ¼ cup of dried fruit. Citrus fruits, melons and berries are all excellent sources of vitamin C and provide other vitamins, such as folate, and minerals, such as potassium. Try to pick these for at least half of your fruit selections. Other fruits contribute the same nutrients, but in smaller amounts. Deep yellow fruits, like apricots, are great sources of vitamin A.

FOOD GROUP 5

All vegetables contribute fiber and are sources of a variety of nutrients. *Three to five daily servings* are recommended. Think of vegetables as falling into three categories: the dark green or deep yellow vegetables, the starchy vegetables and all the others. The dark green vegetables, such as broccoli, spinach and romaine lettuce, are excellent sources of vitamins A and C, riboflavin, folate, iron and magnesium. They should be eaten several times a week. Deep yellow vegetables, such as carrots, pumpkin and sweet potatoes, are particularly rich in vitamin A. The starchy vegetables, which include dried beans, peas and potatoes, are valuable sources of fiber and contribute vitamin B_6 and folate, iron, magnesium and potassium. Other vegetables, like beets, eggplant and onions, contribute varying amounts of vitamins and minerals.

FOOD GROUP 6

Grains, breads and cereals should play a prominent part in our diets. *Six to 11 daily servings are recommended.* A serving might be a slice of bread, ½ cup of cooked rice or 1 ounce of cold cereal. Whole grain and enriched breads and cereals provide iron, thiamine, riboflavin and niacin. In addition, whole grain products provide folate, magnesium, zinc and dietary fiber. Examples of whole grain products are whole wheat bread, rolls, crackers and pasta, brown rice, bulgur, granola, graham crackers, oatmeal, pumpernickel bread and rye crackers. Enriched grain products include bagels, biscuits, corn bread, corn muffins, cornmeal, crackers, English muffins, farina, French bread, grits, Italian bread, noodles, pancakes, pasta, white rice and some ready-to-eat breakfast cereals. Grain-based foods that have substantial amounts of fat or sweeteners—cakes, pies and cookies—probably belong in Food Group 1, to be eaten in moderation.

NUTRITIONISTS

Mary Archer was seriously ill, but she didn't know it. She thought her fatigue, insatiable thirst and frequent urination might be due to something lacking in her diet. Acting on a friend's referral, she drove to an office complex near her Scottsdale, Arizona, home, and knocked on a door with a sign that read "Nutritionist."

She discussed her ailments with a soft-spoken, bespectacled man in his midthirties. He told Archer that he could diagnose her problem by analyzing her hair. From that analysis, he determined that Archer suffered from "metal toxicity," and the only cure was vitamins. Many vitamins. They could be bought elsewhere, but he recommended his own personal stock—a bit expensive maybe, but they were "pure."

Mary Archer would soon grow much sicker.

Many self-anointed nutritionists in this country lack any credentials or nutritional education, according to Stephen Barrett, M.D., an Allentown, Pennsylvania, psychiatrist and well-known crusader against health fraud. They are, in other words, quacks—who sometimes do a lot of harm. Dr. Barrett suspects that Mary Archer fell victim to such a person.

Archer, a college graduate, 45 years old and extremely articulate, can't explain how it happened, but she agrees she was snookered. Her treatments, she says, wound up costing $235 and "almost my life." Today, two years later, under the care of a physician and a professional dietitian, she's gained back the 40 pounds she had lost during her vitamin "cure," and her diabetes—the problem she *really* had—is under control.

AN EASY PROFESSION TO ENTER

Because of cases such as Archer's, Dr. Barrett says it's high time for the government to step in. At present, he explains, the title nutritionist—unlike physician, or attorney, or even dietitian—is not well defined. In fact, only a handful of states have laws regulating who may hang out a shingle and hawk nutritional advice.

Registered dietitians (nutritionists certified by the American Dietetic Association's Committee on Dietetic Registration) are fighting for laws to discipline the field. They're seeking to restrict licensure to R.D.'s, Ph.D.'s in nutrition, M.D.'s and a few other health professionals; all others would be prohibited from giving nutritional advice.

"I can't buy it," says Stanley A. Jacobson, president of the National Nutritional Foods Association (NNFA). The NNFA is the main opponent of the licensure push in the courts. Citing public protection as *his* goal, Jacobson says that while uncredentialed quacks do some harm, the licensing of dietitians as nutritionists would do even more harm. "Just look at the malnutrition in hospitals today," he says, referring to current laws that say hospitals must employ R.D.'s to help plan meals.

Until the issue is decided, there will be those who'll continue to rake in a profit at the expense of people like Mary Archer. There are the dubious "nutritionists," such as the one she ran across. But the sham doesn't end there.

HOW TO BUY A FANCY TITLE

Over the past years, says Dr. Barrett, an entire industry has arisen to provide "credentials" for the uncredentialed practitioner. The American Association of Nutritional Consultants (AANC) offers a fancy certificate to "professional" members who wish to display their "high standards" on the office wall. The cost is $50. Send your money to the association's Las Vegas address, and they'll send you a certificate—no questions asked.

There are schools, too, providing impressive-sounding certificates. The Nutritionists Institute of America in Kansas City (whose literature boasts that its director "was a premedical student" in college) advertises: "Be a certified nutritionist!" When a *Kansas City Star* reporter investigated the school, he found out just how hard it is to gain admittance: a colleague's dog had his application (and money) readily accepted and, with just a little human help, received a certificate.

The same trick has been played on the AANC

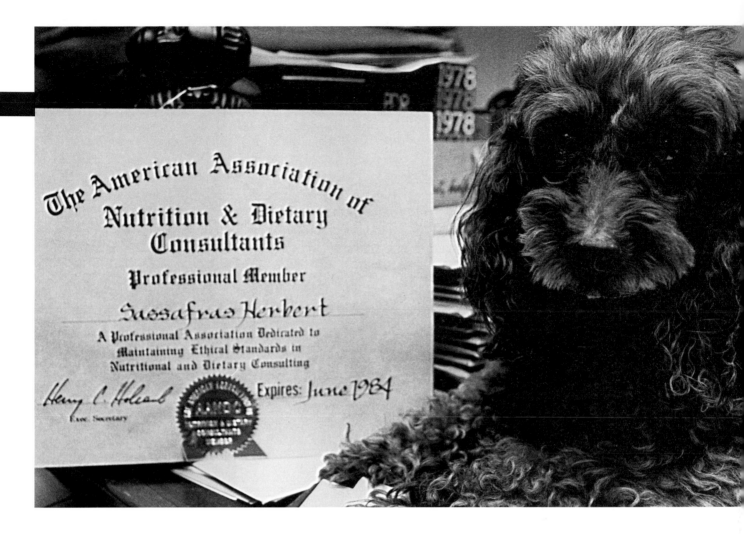

Sassafras Herbert became the subject of a 1984 congressional hearing on health quackery when his owner, Victor Herbert, M.D., J.D., used the poodle's easily won professional affiliation to drive home a point. The American Association of Nutrition and Dietary Consultants has since changed its name, but membership requirements remain the same. Although his membership has expired, Sassafras still has a great interest in nutrition — especially when it comes to biscuits and bones.

several times, so that dogs (and even a hamster) have been admitted to "professional" membership. (See the accompanying photograph.)

According to Chloe Dybdahl, a Nutritionists Institute student, getting through the school's curriculum isn't any tougher than getting in. Chloe is wrapping up a $400 correspondence course, which, the school says, means she's nearly qualified to be a nutrition professional. "I learned a lot of the stuff in

second and third grade," says 10-year-old fourth-grader Chloe.

So what can you do to get good nutritional advice in this wacky world of 10-year-old "certified nutritionists," and canine consultants?
● Look for relevant credentials. A nutritionist who is also an R.D., M.D. or Ph.D. is more likely to have a background in nutritional science than someone who is not.
● Ask your family doctor to refer you to an experienced nutritionist.
● Steer clear of anyone who is offering hair analysis, prescribing *and* selling vitamins or—the cutting edge in quackery—using computer-scored questionnaires for diagnosing "nutrient deficiencies," advises Dr. Barrett.

Be particularly careful if you happen to pass through Scottsdale, Arizona, and you bump into a guy who says you've got metal toxicity. "He's still in business," says Archer.

OSTEOPOROSIS

My mother was always taller than me, even after I grew up," says Julia. "Now her back is bent and I can see over her head. I guess that's just a part of getting old."

A bent back is often the most obvious symptom of osteoporosis, the bone-loss disorder that affects 15 to 20 million Americans. In fact, past the age of 65, one out of every four women may have experienced fractures.

But Julia is wrong about osteoporosis, say the experts. Shrunken bones are not a normal part of aging.

To understand just how bones get dangerously thin, you might think of them as a kind of bank, suggests Robert P. Heaney, M.D., author of *Calcium and Common Sense*. Throughout your youth and until your mid-thirties, explains Dr. Heaney, your body normally deposits calcium into

KIDS AND CALCIUM

Drinking milk gives kids a healthy start in life—and may even help in old age, too. University of Pittsburgh researchers found that women who drank milk three times daily as children had higher bone density than those who drank milk less often. That, they say, may protect against osteoporosis later in life.

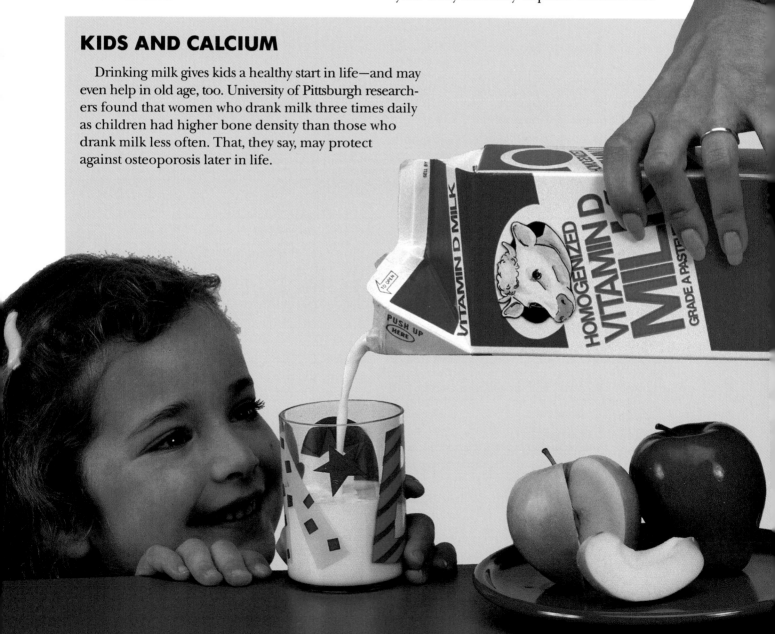

the bones. That's what makes them dense and strong. At the same time, small calcium withdrawals are routinely made to make sure that there is enough calcium circulating in the blood so that the heart can beat properly, the muscles can contract and blood can clot.

By the late thirties, though, both men and women make fewer calcium deposits in the bone bank, partly because we become less able to absorb calcium from food. Women have an even tougher time if, for example, they have had their ovaries removed or have gone through menopause. These women aren't producing enough estrogen (a hormone) to enable the body to use calcium efficiently. The calcium-deficit problem appears to be most pronounced for Caucasian women of slight build who drink or smoke and whose mothers have osteoporosis.

What happens when the body gets too little calcium? The bone bank gets robbed, and osteoporosis takes over. "Bones may provide the rest of the body with adequate calcium, but they wind up sacrificing their own supply," Dr. Heaney says.

CALCIUM FOR A STRONG SPINE

How can you prevent a bent back in old age? Do what your mother told you as a kid: Drink your milk. "That's one way you can build up your bone bank and possibly reduce the risk of osteoporosis," notes Dr. Heaney.

You'll need to consume at least 1,000 milligrams of calcium each day to maintain an adequate calcium balance, suggests B. Lawrence Riggs, M.D., who is associated with the Mayo Clinic. And you can get *more* than that amount just by pouring skim milk on your cereal at breakfast, lunching on a cup of yogurt and pouring a Swiss cheese sauce over your dinner vegetable.

These foods will do the most good if you also exercise. Be sure the milk you drink has been fortified with vitamin D, which helps your body absorb calcium. Limit your intake of caffeine and sodium-laden foods—they speed the loss of calcium from your body.

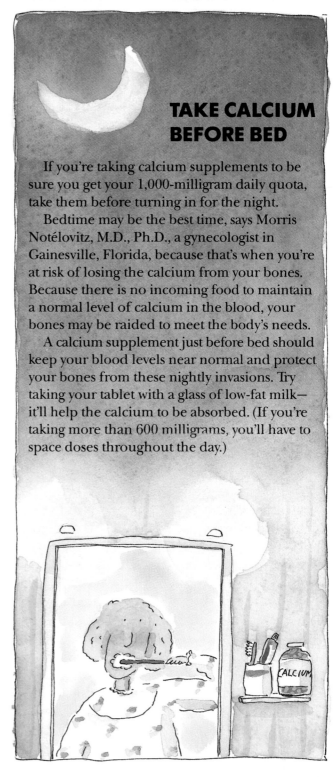

TAKE CALCIUM BEFORE BED

If you're taking calcium supplements to be sure you get your 1,000-milligram daily quota, take them before turning in for the night.

Bedtime may be the best time, says Morris Notélovitz, M.D., Ph.D., a gynecologist in Gainesville, Florida, because that's when you're at risk of losing the calcium from your bones. Because there is no incoming food to maintain a normal level of calcium in the blood, your bones may be raided to meet the body's needs.

A calcium supplement just before bed should keep your blood levels near normal and protect your bones from these nightly invasions. Try taking your tablet with a glass of low-fat milk—it'll help the calcium to be absorbed. (If you're taking more than 600 milligrams, you'll have to space doses throughout the day.)

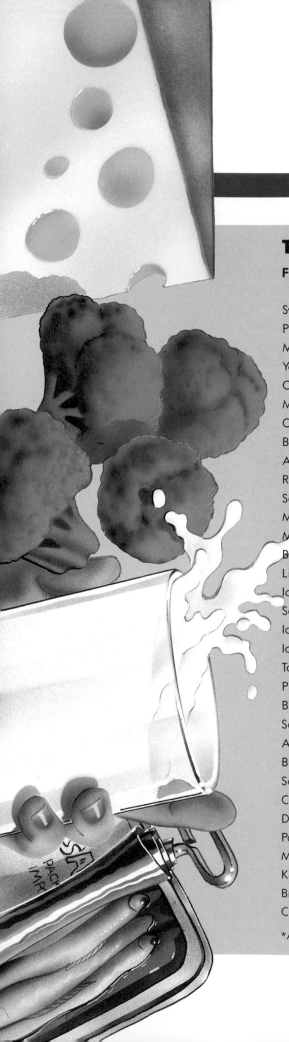

THE BEST FOOD SOURCES OF CALCIUM

FOOD	PORTION	CALCIUM (MG)
Swiss cheese (LS)	2 oz.	544
Provolone cheese	2 oz.	428
Monterey Jack cheese	2 oz.	424
Yogurt, low-fat* (LS)	1 cup	415
Cheddar cheese	2 oz.	408
Muenster cheese	2 oz.	406
Colby cheese	2 oz.	388
Brick cheese	2 oz.	382
American cheese	2 oz.	348
Ricotta cheese, part skim	½ cup	337
Sardines, Atlantic, drained solids*	3 oz.	322
Milk, skim* (LF, LS)	1 cup	302
Mozzarella cheese	2 oz.	294
Buttermilk*	1 cup	285
Limburger cheese	1 cup	282
Ice milk, soft-serve* (LF, LS)	1 cup	274
Salmon, sockeye, with bones* (LS)	3 oz.	203
Ice cream*	1 cup	176
Ice milk* (LF, LS)	1 cup	176
Tofu (LF, LS)	3 oz.	174
Pizza, cheese	⅛ of 14"	144
Blackstrap molasses (LF)	1 Tbsp.	137
Soy flour, defatted	½ cup	120
Almonds, unblanched* (LS)	¼ cup	94
Broccoli, cooked* (LF, LS)	½ cup	89
Soybeans, cooked* (LS)	½ cup	88
Collards, cooked (LF, LS)	½ cup	74
Dandelion greens, cooked	½ cup	73
Parmesan cheese	1 Tbsp.	69
Mustard greens, cooked (LF, LS)	½ cup	52
Kale, cooked (LF, LS)	½ cup	47
Broccoli, raw* (LF, LS)	1 cup	42
Chick-peas, cooked (LS)	½ cup	40

*Also high in potassium.   LF = low-fat.   LS = low-sodium.

OSTEOPOROSIS
A DAY OF INTENSIVE HEALING

A.M.

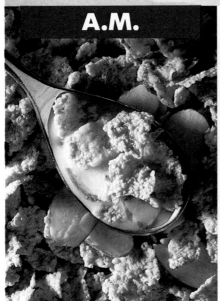

Orange
Whole grain cereal with
  almonds
Skim milk

NOON

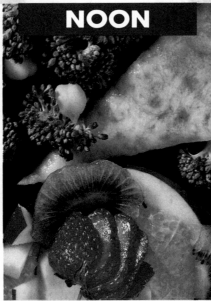

New England clam
  chowder
Two slices pizza
Broccoli and chick-pea
  salad with yogurt
  dressing
Fresh fruit pieces with
  sunflower seeds and
  raisins
Carbonated water

P.M.

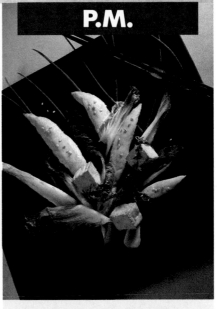

Stir-fried chicken, bok choy,
  tofu and sesame seeds
Steamed collard greens
  with lemon and vinegar
Whole wheat molasses
  muffin
Buttermilk

DISASTER PLATE

Fish fillet or sticks with
  ketchup
Mixed vegetables (peas
  and carrots)

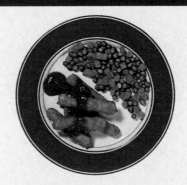

To fight osteoporosis, you
need lots and lots of calcium.
How does this meal add
up? Fish sticks and mixed
vegetables—even a mixture
containing corn, green snap
beans and limas—offer very
little calcium.

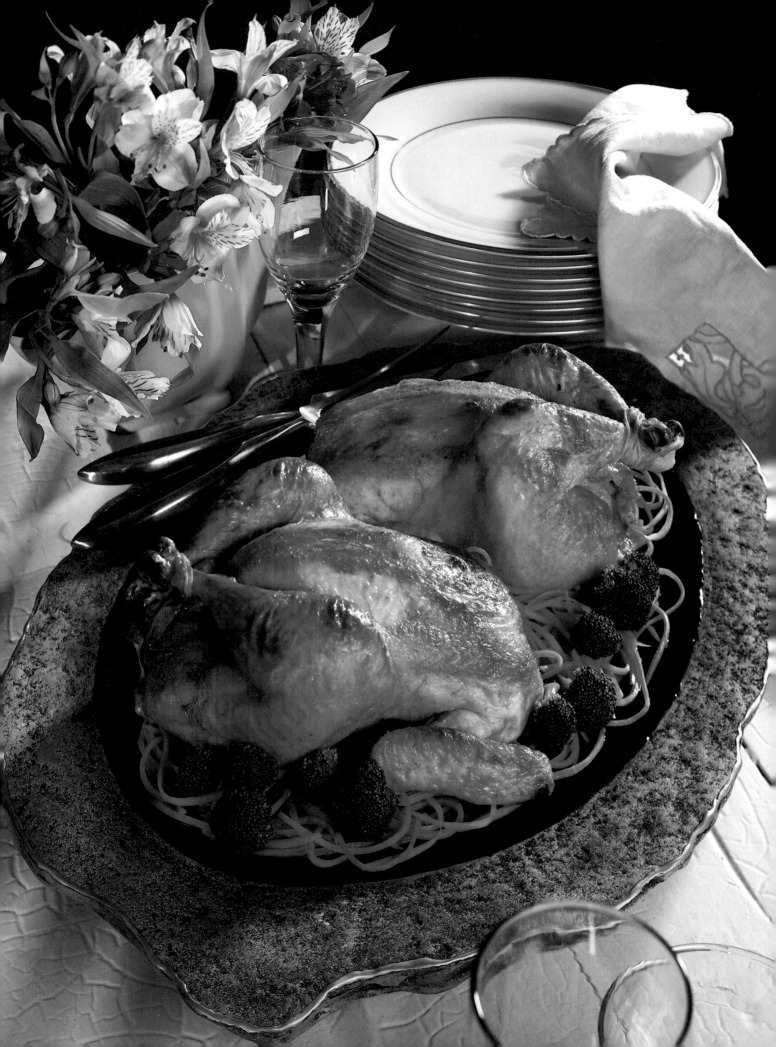

Calcium, calcium, calcium. That's a key word when it comes to preventing osteoporosis, and these three recipes offer significant amounts of this essential nutrient. While yogurt and Swiss cheese are obvious high-calcium choices, salmon and kale are note-worthy sources as well.

YOGURT DIPS AND DRESSINGS

For each of these dips and dressings, mix ⅔ cup plain yogurt and the listed ingredients in a medium-size bowl.

1   tsp. curry powder
1   tsp. paprika
½   tsp. ground cumin
½   tsp. ground coriander

Use as a dressing to rub into chicken before roasting.

¼   cup finely minced smoked salmon or turkey
¼   cup seeded chopped cucumber
     Pinch of fresh dill

Serve with crudités or crackers.

1   peach, chopped
1   Tbsp. maple syrup
     Pinch of freshly grated nutmeg

Serve on waffles, pancakes or hot cereal.

2   Tbsp. prepared horseradish
1   Tbsp. minced fresh chives
¼   cup finely minced red onions

Serve with hot or cold roast beef or as a topping for baked potatoes.

1   cup tomato puree
1   tsp. dillweed

Serve with cold poached salmon or other fish.

SALMON SALAD WITH ALMONDS AND BOK CHOY

10   to 12 bok choy leaves
1   can (8 oz.) red salmon
⅓   cup chopped bok choy ribs
2   scallions, minced
¼   cup sliced almonds
3   Tbsp. plain yogurt
1   Tbsp. crumbled blue cheese

Arrange bok choy leaves on a serving platter. Drain salmon and place in a medium-size bowl. Add bok choy ribs, scallions and almonds and toss carefully so salmon doesn't crumble too much. Gently place salmon mixture on platter.

In a small bowl, combine yogurt and blue cheese. Drizzle over salmon and serve.

Yield: 4 servings

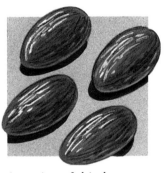

A serving of dried, unblanched almonds can provide as much calcium as a serving of cottage cheese.

ENCHILADAS WITH SWISS CHEESE AND KALE

4   corn tortillas
½   cup finely chopped kale
2   scallions, minced
½   cup shredded Swiss cheese
2   tsp. olive oil
½   cup tomato sauce or puree
     Grated Swiss cheese
     Minced fresh parsley

Preheat a well-seasoned cast-iron skillet over medium-high heat. (Or use a nonstick skillet, but don't preheat.)

Lay out tortillas on counter and sprinkle with equal amounts of kale, scallions and cheese. Roll up each tortilla and press in filling with back of a spoon.

When skillet is hot, add oil, then place enchiladas seam-side down in skillet. Pour tomato sauce or puree over enchiladas and bring to a boil. Reduce heat and simmer for about 5 minutes, basting frequently.

Place enchiladas on a serving platter and square off sides with a spatula. Sprinkle with cheese and parsley and serve hot.

Yield: 4 servings

Leafy greens like kale also offer good amounts of bone-building calcium.

Roasted Chicken Made with Yogurt Dressing

OVERWEIGHT

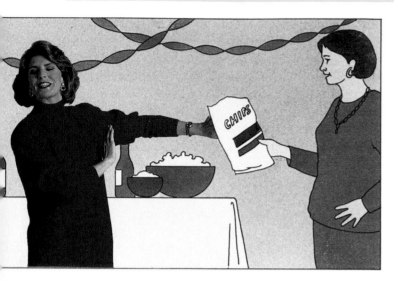

Although dieting represents a big problem for many people, sometimes even little changes can cut it down to size. Who, for example, would think that switching brands of ice cream can save you calories? Well, it can. Go for the inexpensive Brand X—it has less fat in it.

Here are some more simple dietary changes that pack big results:

• Go grocery shopping on a full stomach. Nacho chips, doughnuts and other tempters won't have half the allure they would if you hunted through those aisles hungry.

• Take only a limited amount of money to the grocery store as an extra reinforcement against buying high-calorie foods.

• Don't eat foods out of their original containers. You may think you're having "just a tad," but you'll probably consume more than if you had dished out the food in a measured portion. Better yet, don't bring your "weakness food" into the house in the first place. Present yourself with the hassle of going to the store for single servings.

• Don't skip meals. You'll only overeat later.

• Use good plate psychology. Don't use place settings with intense colors such as violet, lime green, bright yellow or bright blue; they're thought to stimulate the appetite. The same goes for primitive-

Learn that it's okay to say, "No, thank you" when other people offer you food.

looking pewter and wooden plates. Instead, appease your appetite with elegant place settings in darker colors. Choose plates with broad decorative borders and a slightly "bowled" design. You can fit less food on them.

• Police your eating speed by putting your fork down between bites. The slower you eat, the faster you'll feel full.

• Establish a time-out routine halfway through your meals. One trick: Put a large pot of water on the stove when you sit down to eat. When it boils (in about 10 or 15 minutes), get up and make a pot of herb tea. When you go back to the table, you probably won't feel like eating much more.

• Use whipped or softened butter or margarine. You'll spread the flavor around using a lot less than if it were hard and you had to scrape it on.

Invite your spouse or housemate into the kitchen with you when you're preparing meals and cleaning up to keep you from sampling as you go.

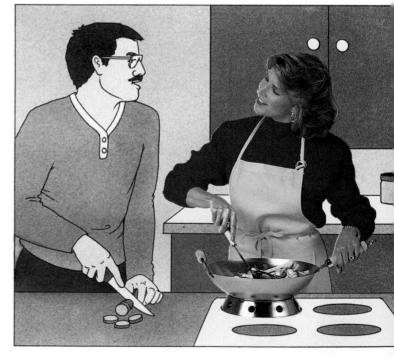

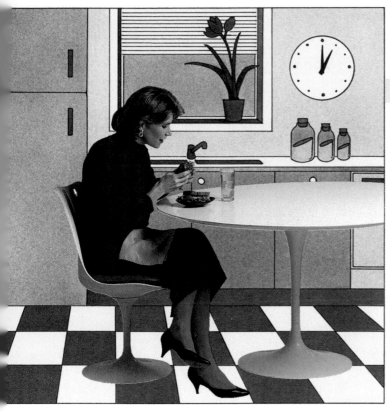

Eat only at scheduled times at scheduled places.

• Drink no-calorie sparkling waters when you're out, instead of alcoholic beverages.

• Remove food stashed in inappropriate places. Get the candy bars out of your desk drawer, and remove the nut bowl from the coffee table.

Shop from a list of necessities. Allow yourself only one purchase that wasn't preplanned.

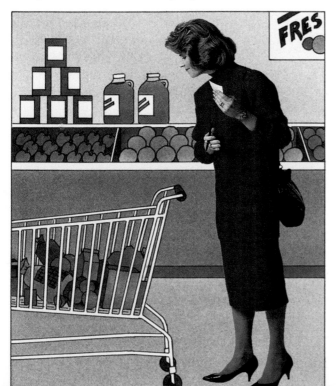

• Have someone else serve you and ask for smaller portions.

• Chew each bite of food at least ten times to really taste it and to make yourself eat more slowly.

• Leave the table as soon as you have finished eating, instead of lingering over the last bites.

• Don't eat everything on your plate (unless you're having steamed vegetables and fish or an equally good-for-you meal).

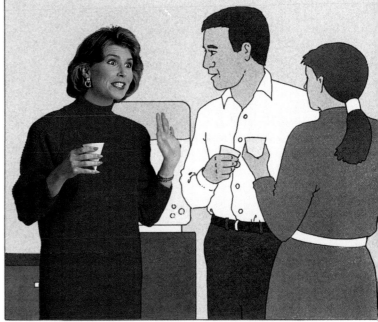

Hold a conference and explain your weight-loss wish to family, friends or doughnut-bearing co-workers. Ask them to understand if you turn down their dinners or candy.

• Get rid of those degrading signs and pictures on your refrigerator—no 300-pound women in bikinis or pink pigs on beach blankets to shame you into not eating. Your willpower will be stronger from encouragement, not belittlement.

• Set a realistic goal for yourself. "Take it one day at a time and don't punish yourself for slipping," says Suzann Johnson, a registered dietitian and a nutritionist with Weight Watchers International. "You'll be more successful if you remember to be your own best friend."

NATHAN PRITIKIN

ven his death was a convincing argument for his way of life.

"His arteries were amazingly clean for a man of his age [69]," says Jeffrey Hubbard, M.D., an Albany pathologist who performed the autopsy on Nathan Pritikin.

While he lived, Nathan Pritikin wrote six books about the theory and practice of the heart-saving diet that bears his name—and that achievement was only part of his relentless, one-man campaign to change the health habits of a nation.

"Basically, all I'm trying to do is wipe out heart disease, hypertension and diabetes in this country," he once said. In his case, that wasn't an overstatement. "He approached his work with missionary zeal," says his son Robert Pritikin, director of the Pritikin Longevity Centers.

Nathan began his mission in 1957, when he was 40 years old. He was told his cholesterol level was 280 and was diagnosed as having heart disease. His doctor put him on a prescription drug for the disease and ordered him not to exert himself—not to walk more than four or five blocks a day, to take a nap in the afternoon and to eliminate strenuous exercise, including bicycle riding and tennis.

FINDING THE THREAD

Needless to say, that advice didn't sit well with Nathan. Instead, he decided to treat his condition—his way.

Robert watched his father methodically go about his task. "My dad had this incredible ability to step away from a personal problem and approach it just like it was a research problem." Nathan was especially methodical when the thing that needed solving involved health.

"He was always interested in health and in being a doctor," Robert says. He read medical journals the way some people read mystery or romance novels—voraciously. And he combined that curiosity, that intensity, with insight.

"My dad's best skill in life was his ability to see a single, unifying principle—an underlying thread—in a very complex array of seemingly disparate and contradictory data. He always said, 'Once you really understand a problem, it's very simple to solve it.' "

The thread appeared in a research study conducted in England after World War II. "He found a top secret study which showed that the heart disease death rate in England dropped during the war, a time at which meat and dairy products were being rationed," says Robert.

And that thread appeared in other studies. "He'd noticed for years that there were populations all over the world who weren't getting heart disease. When he put that information together with what he knew about the results of the rationed diet of England during the war, something clicked—something that led to a decade of research. Ultimately, he found what he believed was the cause of heart disease—diet."

STARTING A REVOLUTION

Today, that conclusion might seem obvious. But in the 1950s—when the high-fat American diet was thought by scientists to be the healthiest in the world, and heart disease was seen as the inevitable

SIX WAYS TO HEALTHY EATING

- Don't eat fats or oils—avoid fatty meats like hamburger and "marbled" steak. Avoid cooking oils, salad oils, vegetable oils and shortening.
- Don't eat dairy products unless they are nonfat (skim).
- Don't eat sugar, honey, molasses, pies, cakes and pastries.
- Don't eat salt or salty foods.
- Don't eat food high in cholesterol, such as organ meats, skin, shellfish and egg yolks.
- Don't drink coffee or tea (except herbal teas).

(These diet guidelines are adapted from Nathan Pritikin's book *Live Longer Now.*)

result of aging and stress—that conclusion was revolutionary. Even bolder was Nathan's decision to act on the basis of his new theory.

His first step was to find a diet that would drastically reduce his blood level of cholesterol. Reviewing studies of populations that had low death rates from heart disease and diabetes, he considered their various diets. He adapted the basics of these diets into his own life. He then kept meticulous records of his own dietary cholesterol intake and his blood levels of the fat. He then settled on a diet that consisted of 10 percent fat, 15 percent protein and 75 percent complex carbohydrates, such as whole grains, vegetables and fruits. By the summer of 1958, his cholesterol level had dropped almost by half, to 160. In August of 1959 it was at 155. By the spring of 1960 it had fallen to 120.

His second step—again based on a careful reading of scientific literature—was to add exercise to his personal program.

His third step was onto a treadmill. In February, 1966, Nathan took a stress test, in which he ran on a treadmill while being hooked up to an electrocardiograph (EKG), a machine that shows whether the heart is normal. The result: no trace of heart disease.

"I can't tell you how elated I was," he wrote. "I knew I was finished with my heart problem. From that point on, I knew I would try to convert everyone in the world to a new way of living." His dedication led him to a clinical trial and, later, to personal work with those who needed his help.

THE PRITIKIN LONGEVITY CENTERS

One of the early groups of "converts" were the 16 people—heart patients and some of their spouses—who participated in the first month-long program of the Pritikin Longevity Center, which opened in January 1976, at a Howard Johnson's Motor Lodge near Nathan's hometown of Santa Barbara, California. They were so ill that Nathan had to help them inside. "From the start of the project," Robert says, "Dad was absolutely convinced that we would show some reversal in their heart disease, that we'd get

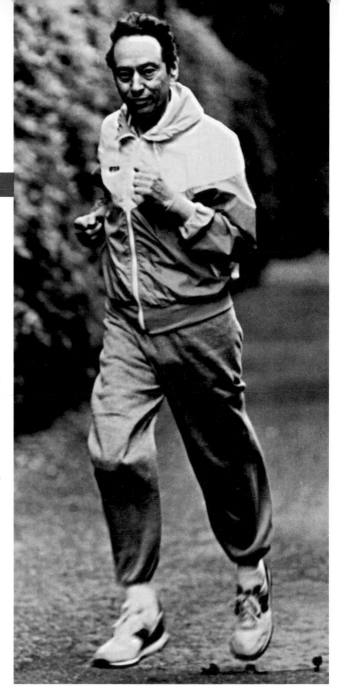

Nathan Pritikin made exercise an integral part of the Pritikin Program. At the centers, the medically supervised exercise programs are individually geared to the participant. Once eating habits are changed and the person gets into good shape, with cholesterol, stress, and blood-pressure levels in a safe range, jogging is encouraged.

them off their medication and stabilize their risk factors."

And that's just what happened. At the end of the 30 days of exercise and low-fat eating, patients who could barely walk when they arrived were walking 10 to 15 miles a day. As a group, their blood cholesterol dropped an average of 25 percent. And the majority were medication free.

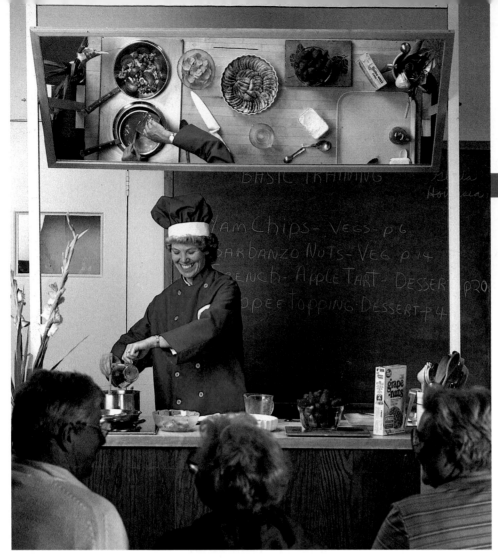

At the Pritikin Longevity Centers, attendees learn the fine art of healthy cooking. Here the instructor shows how to prepare foods deliciously — without using salt and without adding fat.

Since 1976, over 40,000 people have participated in programs at various Pritikin Longevity Centers (which are now housed in private facilities in California, Florida and Pennsylvania). But people who attend them go through pretty much the same program as the original "Pritikin Pioneers."

A PRITIKIN DAY

"The Pritikin Program revolves around dieting, exercising and going to lectures," says Steve Billone, program director at the Longevity Center in Miami Beach.

"The people get up early and do some easy walking or stretching, then eat a breakfast such as oatmeal and whole wheat bread. From 8:00 to 9:00 they go to a lecture about medicine, lifestyles, nutrition or exercise. Then they exercise for 40 minutes, followed by a snack break, then another lecture. Lunch is next, followed by an hour-long cooking

class, then another exercise break. In the late afternoon, there are more lectures. So they're kept busy." So are the physicians who supervise them.

John Tumola, M.D., a cardiologist and medical director of the Downingtown, Pennsylvania, center, says he examines people when they start the program, as they're going through it and when they leave. He *sees* the changes. "They come with high blood pressure; they leave with it at normal levels. They come on medication; they leave off of it. And the majority

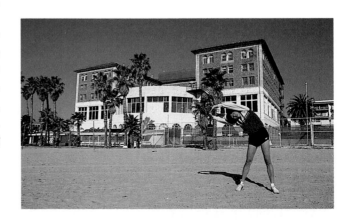

Those who attend the Pritikin Center in Santa Barbara have the wonderful option of exercising on the beach.

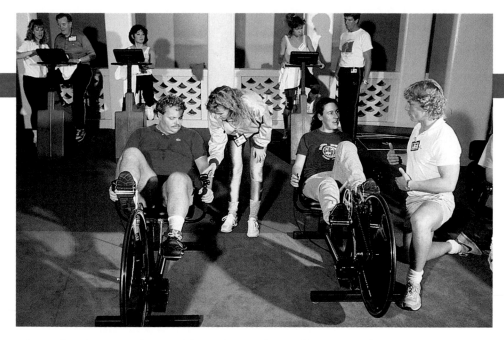

The Pritikin staff carefully monitors these bicyclists to make sure that they get the benefits of exercise, without putting too much strain on the heart.

of people who come here with angina end up taking less medication and experiencing less angina pain."

A PRITIKIN SUCCESS STORY

Statistics don't stop eating quiche. They don't exercise, and they don't go to lectures. People do. John Parent is a person who has been through the Pritikin Program. He knows what the statistics and research say, but more importantly, he knew how he felt at the start: "I was a mess. I weighed 311. On a good day, my cholesterol was around 318. I didn't exercise. I was a heart attack waiting to happen."

So the 48-year-old president and chief executive officer of a company that owned a Dairy Queen and a few Donut Huts dunked himself into a 13-day Pritikin Program. Four weeks later, the tale of the tape showed a new man. "I lost 32 pounds, my cholesterol was cut by a third to 207, and I was even exercising on a bicycle for an hour a day every morning. I felt great."

He felt so good, in fact, that he decided that what he had learned at the program should be shared with others. So he started his own "program." "At the restaurants we stopped adding salt to the french fries, and the customers tell us they like that better. I'm even starting to have salad bars available now." Nathan would be proud.

Mealtime is fun time. It allows people to socialize and to compare notes on their fitness progress.

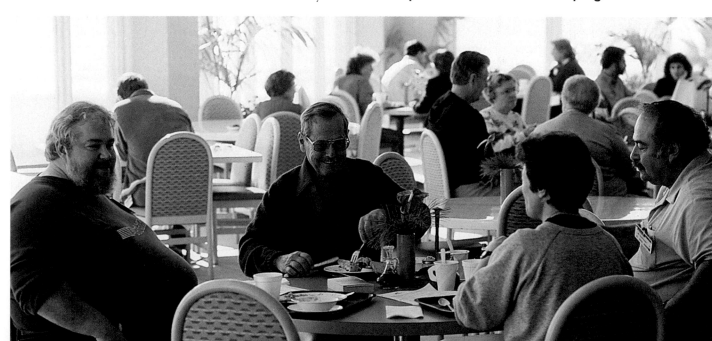

THE PSYCHOLOGY OF INTENSIVE HEALING

A special diet, at least in theory, is like love. It should last forever.

But when salted peanuts are your passion and you've been told "no salt," your special diet may seem more like a prison term than a happy marriage. Here are some tried-and-true techniques to help you live with your diet. Try these tips on for size.

Buddy up. Most healing diets are also *good* diets—good for people in general. If yours is such a regimen, enlist the help of your family. With everyone on your low-sodium (or low-fat or high-fiber) diet, you won't be left drooling while others eat your former favorite dishes.

"Your success rate is much higher if you get support from the family. No question about it," adds Walt Funk, lifestyle counselor of the health division at Pennsylvania's West Chester State University.

Play down perfection. Many people tend to apply their goal-oriented ways to succeeding at their special diets. But in a special diet, says Funk, it's not whether you win or lose. It's how you play the game.

By focusing on a goal—say it's achieving a cholesterol level of 180—we miss out on the process, and the process of the whole behavior change has to be enjoyable. Besides, "as soon as people say, 'I've won,' they want to give themselves a reward—that is, eating all the wrong things," says Funk. Instead of conquering your diet, focus instead on one day at a time. Don't think you've failed because you were seduced by gelato while on a low-cholesterol diet. And remember that, once made, these changes will serve you for the rest of your life.

Focus on the big picture. If you're on a diet to control hypertension, you'll have a better shot at

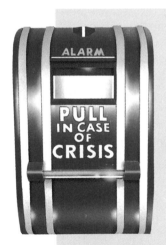

HELP!

Here are some strategies to get you through those short-term diet-threatening emergencies.

Play with your food. You want to be a polite guest, but you want to stick to your healing diet. "Do two things," says counselor Walt Funk. "Eat small portions of those foods that come as close as possible to meeting your new dietary requirements and learn to move the food around on your plate. Like the teetotaler who drinks club soda with a twist of lemon, you fit into the social situation without making yourself obvious," he says.

Avoid the terrible too's. Try to avoid becoming too bored, too tired, too angry and so on. "It's these extremes that usually cause us to backslide," says Funk.

Eat before you go out. Don't go to social gatherings hungry. "Load up on some healthy food before you go," says

psychologist Michael R. Lowe, Ph.D.

Launch a preemptive strike. Say you're on a special diet and your client wants to discuss the big contract over a three-martini lunch. What's the best way to balance his plans with your dietary needs? Let your client know ahead of time that you are on a special diet. "Don't wait until you sit down with that person, then order a salad," says Funk. By letting him know ahead of time, he's not surprised by your food choices and you preempt his chance to wheedle you into "just having a couple."

Mind over matter. Mom keeps pushing her peanut butter pie, and you keep pushing back. No matter who tries to sabotage your diet, the most effective remedy is simple persistence, says Dr. Lowe. Just say no. And keep saying it.

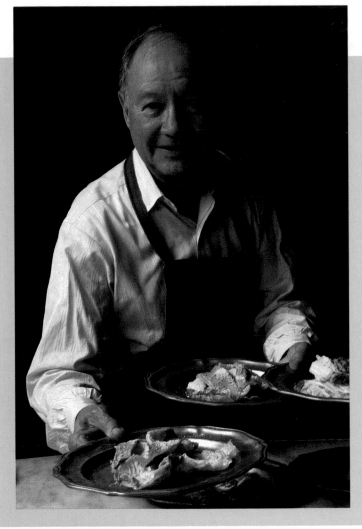

staying on it if you view it as just one part of your overall plan for better health.

So while you're concentrating on your intensive healing diet, you also may want to consider other lifestyle changes, like an exercise program (consult your doctor first, of course). Take a look at the role stress plays in your life and take steps to rein in your snarling anxieties.

Exercise in particular plays a central role in the dietary advice of Kelly D. Brownell, Ph.D., codirector of the Obesity Clinic at the University of Pennsylvania. And make no mistake: Exercise is not just for people who need to lose weight. It's for people on all kinds of diets who need to *gain* a healthier lifestyle.

Disarm your dietary triggers. What makes a person on a special diet for high blood pressure devour a bag of salty microwave popcorn? Hunger? Television commercials? Loneliness? Anxiety? No matter what the cause, root it out, says Funk.

Often we're tripped up by those triggers. So if you know you only break out the popcorn when you're watching a football game on the tube, work hard to develop a different response.

Consider positive alternatives. Many people never realize the long-term benefits of healing diets because they see their diets as a burden. They think negatively, as in, "I must *stop* eating cholesterol-laden foods or I have to *avoid* salt."

Successful dieters, on the other hand, have a Pollyanna streak—a sensible one. Instead of dwelling on all the bad things that they must avoid, they concentrate on positive alternatives.

"No one should be confined to a lifetime of eating monotonous foods," says Michael R. Lowe, Ph.D., director of the Weight Management Program for Temple University Medical Practices in Philadelphia. "There are a lot of low-calorie, healthier, more interesting ways of eating, but you have to look for them. Develop an active interest in alternative eating. Go to restaurants that offer healthier cooking."

RECUPERATION

The city sparkles in the sunlight, a monument to man's ability to shape the world to fit his needs.

The hospital, surrounded by green lawns and clean concrete walkways, is a monument of a different sort. It marks the ability of man's mind to throw up barricades and fight the armies of disease and pestilence.

But on a carefully made-up hospital bed, a casualty of that conflict lies dying. He is a man whose barriers collapsed under the assault and who is paying the ultimate price.

The irony of it: The dying man was a scion of his society, educated at the best schools, employed near the pinnacle of his profession and with access to the best medical advice available. Admitted for routine surgery, he should be well on his way to recovery. He's dying instead, the victim of a hospital-acquired infection. At the time of his admission, he had an underlying mild but chronic illness. He had lost his appetite and had lost weight. And the reason he succumbed to this infection was malnutrition.

THE SITUATION

"It's hard to look at a well-to-do, trim person and realize that he may actually be suffering from malnutrition, but that's often the case," says George Blackburn, M.D., director of Nutrition Support Services at New England Deaconess Hospital and associate professor of surgery at Harvard Medical School.

"You ask yourself, how can that be? Well, consider one of my patients: A woman who can buy and get anything she wants to eat but has a chronic illness that led to a deficient diet. To make matters worse, she also has a sensitive stomach and some food fetishes.

"She came here for surgery, but the fact is we *can't* operate: She's so poorly nourished she would be at very high risk, so that's what we have to fix first—her diet."

Malnutrition is a problem for people facing surgery or experiencing illness simply because it has a direct effect on their ability to combat the metabolic stresses involved. The malnourished person, whether a poor mother in Appalachia or a pampered socialite fresh in from the Caribbean, could be less able to fight off infection or repair tissue damaged by disease or surgery.

"The risk is significant," Dr. Blackburn says. "Not everyone admitted to the hospital faces it, but I'd estimate that between 10 to 15 percent of the population in this country is suffering from what we would define as malnutrition." The chronically ill and those who are elderly and infirm are at highest risk.

Based on the results of Dr. Blackburn's research and involvement in Boston-area hospitals, he estimates that nutritional support can reduce the risks posed by malnutrition. Hospitals that use preadmission screening and *active* efforts to ensure that people eat what they need to remedy their deficiencies will cut the risk of death or serious complications by at least half when treating the following conditions:
- Fistulas (abnormal passages between hollow internal organs or the surface of the body)—10 percent, down from a norm of 50 percent.
- Regional enteritis (an inflammation, usually in a section of the small intestine)—5 percent, down from a rate of 30 percent.
- Pancreatitis (inflammation of the pancreas)—5 percent, down from 20 percent.
- Cancer surgery—25 percent, down from a grim 75 percent.

THE SOLUTION

What do these statistics mean for you? They mean that there's a great deal you can do as an individual to make sure that your doctor's expertise doesn't go for naught. Dr. Blackburn's program for making sure your hospital stay doesn't last any longer than it absolutely has to is short and sweet.

"Realize that improving your nutritional status is something you have to do in partnership with the medical community. We have the expertise to tell you where you're starting from, and you need to know that. So go to a clinic—this is a situation that's difficult for a single doctor to handle properly—and have your diet and health evaluated."

Given that, Dr. Blackburn suggests the following steps to bolster your body against the battering of disease or injury.

Eat right. "But if you have no appetite or a poor diet, a good vitamin and mineral supplement isn't a bad idea if you're risking serious illness or prolonged hospitalization. It's a way to make sure you're getting the 40 micronutrients we all need. The trace minerals (zinc, selenium and magnesium, for example) are very important to immune-system function," he says.

Get regular, good exercise. "This can have a tremendous impact on your resistance to infection and in optimizing your recovery. Brisk walking is ideal. Walk five to seven times a week, aiming for a minimum of 2½ miles each time, at a rate of 15 to 16 minutes per mile."

Get regular checkups. "It's peculiar, but the same people who have their car tuned up every three months don't think twice about going years without having *themselves* looked at," says Dr. Blackburn.

HOSPITAL FOOD FLUNKS

Suppose you spent two weeks in the hospital, recovering from a disease. Under medical care, watched over by nurses and fed meals planned by a professional nutritionist, you'd expect to emerge not only recovered but also well nourished.

Not necessarily. A survey of 3,047 patients in 33 hospitals was performed in Chicago. As the graph at right shows, 58% of those admitted were already in a poor nutritional state. The other 42% were considered "acceptable."

Another study showed that 75 percent of those hospitalized for two weeks or more had a poorer nutritional status than when they were admitted.

Says Harvard's George Blackburn, M.D., who has examined the malnutrition problem in American hospitals: "Approximately one out of six American hospital patients today does not benefit from proper nutritional care," he says.

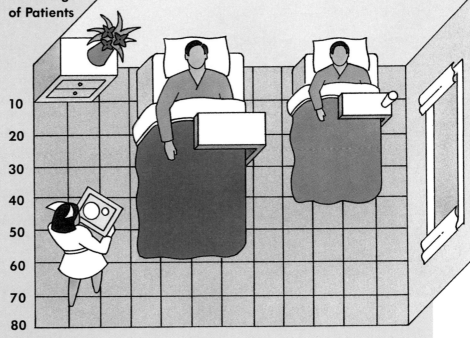

Percentage of Patients

10 20 30 40 50 60 70 80

■ Patients at Nutritional Risk

□ Patients Not at Nutritional Risk

SIPPY AND THE BLAND DIET

INSIPID: *adj. 1. lacking taste or savor. 2. lacking in qualities that interest, stimulate or challenge.*

No, the word "insipid" was not coined to describe the work of Bertram W. Sippy, M.D. But don't try to tell that to people whose ulcers were treated with some form of the Sippy diet. They're the folks who gave up spicy delicacies for custard and oatmeal, the ones who traded in chili dogs for soft-boiled eggs and dry martinis for warm milk.

Now it turns out that drinking milk may *not* be a good thing to do for an ulcer. And there is no scientific evidence whatsoever that a bland diet helps an ulcer heal.

Whoa! Wait a minute. Before all you current and former ulcer sufferers burn Dr. Sippy in effigy, let's take a look at the man's historical contribution.

ULCER TREATMENT REVOLUTION

Born in 1866, Dr. Sippy developed an extensive medical practice around the turn of the century in Chicago. His landmark article on the treatment of gastric and duodenal ulcers through dietary means rather than surgery was published in 1915 in the *Journal of the American Medical Association.* The treatment of ulcers would never again be the same.

"From our present perspective, it is hard to imagine the confusion and conflict surrounding the treatment of ulcers that existed at the end of the 19th century," says Geoffrey Zucker, M.D., a Massachusetts gastroenterologist. Before Dr. Sippy's work changed things, the treatment of choice for most ulcers was surgery, says Dr. Zucker, who has written articles about Dr. Sippy for professional publications.

Dr. Sippy didn't come up with anything really new in terms of treatment. But he did recognize the importance of neutralizing stomach acid with diet, according to Dr. Zucker.

Milk was a natural choice for Dr. Sippy to make, but far from a revolutionary one. As far back as Gaius Pliny (A.D. 23–79), ass's milk was prescribed for people suffering from ulcer pain. Moreover, bland diets and frequent feedings were also familiar ulcer treatments in Dr. Sippy's day. It was what Dr. Sippy did with all those things that counted.

Walter Palmer, M.D., 91, a retired gastroenterologist who interned under Dr. Sippy in 1923, describes the legendary physician as an inspiration to both his patients and his fellow doctors.

"He would have made a wonderful preacher," says Dr. Palmer. "He was a salesman. He had a good article to sell, and he sold it to people who needed help because they had stomach distress, a tummyache."

Dr. Sippy sold his patients on the idea of sticking to a strict dietary regimen that required no small amount of discipline to follow. And he sold fellow physicians on the idea of trying this mode of treatment before resorting to surgery.

DR. SIPPY HAD THE RIGHT IDEA

Dr. Sippy's reasoning was scientifically sound, according to Dr. Zucker. He realized that pain was due to the action of stomach acid on the ulcer and that the key to eliminating pain and promoting healing was to neutralize the stomach acid. He ordered bed rest for his patients (thereby reducing stress) and prescribed hourly feedings of a mixture of milk and cream. He removed digestive acid from their stomachs during the night by means of a tube.

These days, digestive acids are neutralized with drugs. And milk is no longer prescribed because while it is a great buffer of stomach acid, it also *stimulates* its secretion. Also, milk and cream are high in fat.

"No one knew about cholesterol and triglycerides in 1915," says Dr. Zucker. "That's why your grandparents died of clogged arteries."

Dr. Sippy himself died while still in his fifties, probably of heart disease. But his legacy lives on. His theories about when surgical intervention is necessary are still followed.

"I think his therapy, his thoughts, his theory on the treatment of ulcers are still correct," says Dr. Zucker. "It's not been debunked; it's been improved upon."

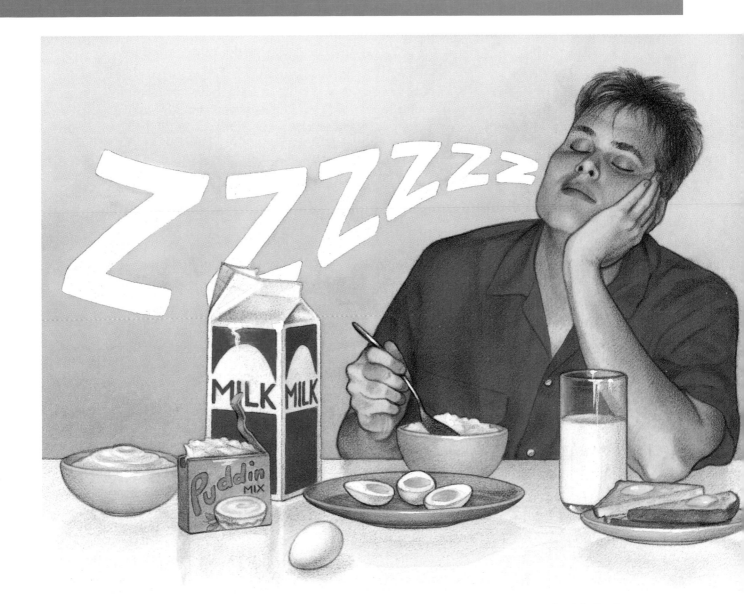

Once upon a time an ulcer diagnosis meant being condemned to one of the ho-hum diets that bore Dr. Sippy's name. Your gustatory pleasures in life would have been severely curtailed.

If you have an ulcer, your doctor these days might give you some medication and tell you that you can eat whatever you want as long as it doesn't cause you any discomfort. And you can thank Dr. Sippy that your ulcer is being treated through nonsurgical means.

Ulcer sufferers being treated with Dr. Bertram Sippy's bland diet dozed over endless repasts of oatmeal, soft-boiled eggs, pureed vegetables and milk. That wasn't just what they had for breakfast—that's what they had for food. Period. And you thought reducing diets were boring?

STROKE

Bang. Your coffee cup shatters as it hits the kitchen floor. Suddenly, the world seems to be moving in slow motion.

You try to pick up the cup with your right hand, but your arm refuses to move. Then you notice the funny, prickly feeling on the right side of your face. Your lower lip feels heavy. Your body starts to droop to the right. Slowly, almost peacefully, everything fades to black.

Life has changed. Normal is out the window, and a new word has suddenly burst into your life. It's called stroke, and it's what you've just experienced. "A stroke is a sudden dysfunction of the brain caused by either a blockage of blood flow or hemorrhage from a burst blood vessel," says Thomas Robertson, M.D., chief of the Cardiac Diseases Branch of the National Institutes of Health. "There is an abrupt, or

sudden, onset of paralysis. The paralysis usually is on one side of the body, but it can affect both sides. It may be followed by a splitting severe headache, then a lapse into unconsciousness."

Sometimes strokes send out advance warnings of what's to come. "Frequently there are so-called small strokes," says Dr. Robertson. "These are episodes of paralysis or numbness that occur and then subside, either within a matter of minutes or in an hour or two. Such warning strokes are certainly evidence that something is wrong, and you should see a physician right away for an evaluation."

WHO IS STRICKEN BY STROKE?

More than two million people in the United States have suffered strokes, with 150,000 people dying from them annually. Stroke is the third leading

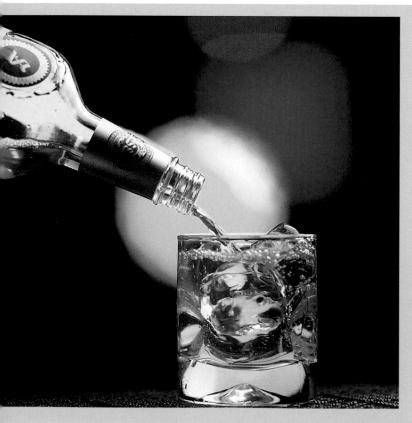

HEAVY DRINKING AND RISK OF STROKE

It seems that if you're a heavy drinker, a hangover may be the least of your problems.

In two recent studies, Jaswinder Gill, research fellow at the Royal Post Graduate Medical School, Hammersmith Hospital, London, found that your chances for having a stroke are much higher if you're a heavy drinker than if you're a teetotaler or a light drinker.

"If you're drinking more than two pints of beer a day, or three or four shots of alcohol a day, every day, seven days a week, you have a four times higher risk of developing a stroke than people who don't drink," he says.

Dr. Gill also found out, though, that "if you're a light drinker, you seem to be somewhat protected from the effects of a stroke."

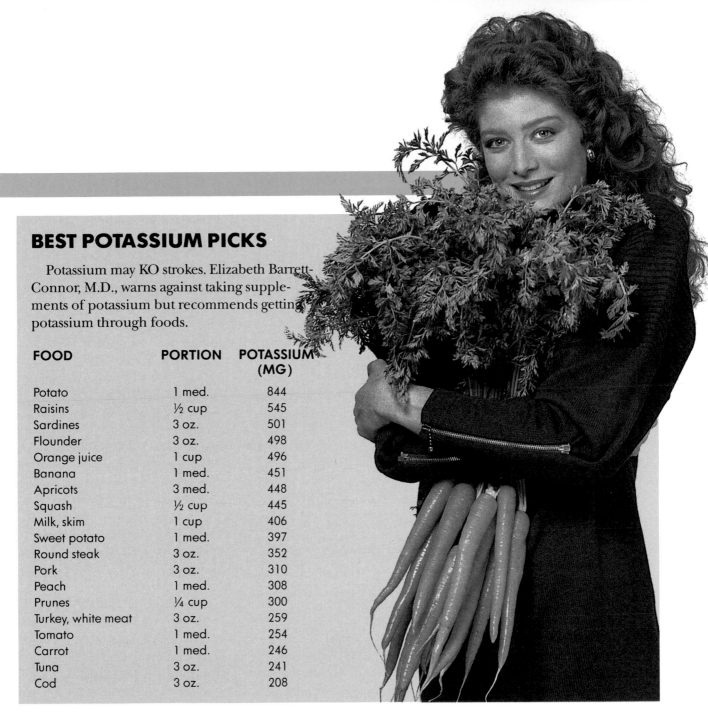

BEST POTASSIUM PICKS

Potassium may KO strokes. Elizabeth Barrett-Connor, M.D., warns against taking supplements of potassium but recommends getting potassium through foods.

FOOD	PORTION	POTASSIUM (MG)
Potato	1 med.	844
Raisins	½ cup	545
Sardines	3 oz.	501
Flounder	3 oz.	498
Orange juice	1 cup	496
Banana	1 med.	451
Apricots	3 med.	448
Squash	½ cup	445
Milk, skim	1 cup	406
Sweet potato	1 med.	397
Round steak	3 oz.	352
Pork	3 oz.	310
Peach	1 med.	308
Prunes	¼ cup	300
Turkey, white meat	3 oz.	259
Tomato	1 med.	254
Carrot	1 med.	246
Tuna	3 oz.	241
Cod	3 oz.	208

cause of death and disability in this country.

The older you are, the more likely it is that you will have a stroke, says James Halsey, M.D., director of the Stroke Research Center at the University of Alabama.

Where you live can also make a difference. Strokes seem to especially favor one region of the country. "The Southeast is where strokes are most common," says Dr. Halsey, "even when you adjust for blood pressure and race. [Blacks are more likely than whites to suffer strokes.] You have a much higher chance of having a stroke if you live in say, Atlanta, than if you live in Denver." Dr. Halsey says it's not known why strokes prefer the Sun Belt to a

Rocky Mountain high, but he also says that research has found three main factors that contribute to stroke.

Hypertension is first on the list. In fact, according to Dr. Halsey, high blood pressure is the single most important factor in causing strokes.

Second, your chances of not having a stroke may go up in smoke. Dr. Halsey says the simple (or not so simple) act of quitting smoking will dramatically reduce the likelihood of ever suffering a stroke.

The third very important factor is your diet. Stroke follows a basic recipe. "It's been known for a long time that there is a strong relationship between high blood cholesterol and stroke," says Dr. Halsey. "We get too much cholesterol in our food and much too much fat, especially saturated fat. We eat too many hamburgers and not enough fish."

These three risk factors can lead to deadly consequences, as Frank Yatsu, M.D., chairman of the Department of Neurology at the University of Texas Medical School at Houston, found out. In a research study of over 4,000 stroke patients, Dr. Yatsu discovered that "95 percent of the people already had risk factors before they had the stroke. Certainly if you have no risk factors, or do away with the ones you have, the risk of having a stroke becomes very small."

Researchers agree that one way to control your risk is to control what's in your diet.

REDUCING YOUR RISKS

Glue up the holes in your salt shaker, or at least retire it from the kitchen table. That action alone could go a long way in reducing your risk of a stroke. For many people, sodium is public enemy number one. "There is little doubt that sodium intake is a contributor to high blood pressure," says Dr. Robertson. "Your blood pressure may decrease once you control your sodium intake."

Another thing to do is lean toward a less fatty diet. "The basic rule," says Dr. Halsey, "is to reduce your overall consumption of fat while replacing saturated with unsaturated fats."

And as recent research studies are showing, aim for a diet high in potassium. Potatoes, it seems, may mash your chances for having a stroke. So may bananas, tomatoes or any other potassium-rich food, according to Elizabeth Barrett-Connor, M.D., chairman of the Department of Community and Family Medicine at the University of California, San Diego. In a 12-year study, she divided 859 men and women into three groups according to the amount of potassium in their diets. The categories ranged from low to average to high amounts of potassium intake. At the study's end, those people in the low-intake group had the highest number of stroke-associated deaths.

Those in the other groups did remarkably better. "People who ate high levels of potassium seemed to have no strokes at all," says Dr. Barrett-Connor. The study also found that a 400-milligram increase in daily potassium intake was associated with a 40 percent reduction in risk. "Practically," Dr. Barrett-Connor adds, "what we're saying is, by just adding an extra serving of fruit or vegetable a day, people could in fact protect themselves against having a stroke."

This increase in potassium consumption might not be a revolutionary idea, but as one researcher suggests, it may be an evolutionary one.

PREHISTORIC PROTECTION

Potassium helps to prevent strokes by protecting certain key cells from injury, says Louis Tobian, M.D., of the University of Minnesota School of Medicine. He found in tests on laboratory animals that a diet high in potassium lowered the stroke rate by 91 percent. "A high-potassium diet protects the endothelial cells, the cells that line the blood vessels, from the injury of high blood pressure," says Dr. Tobian. "By protecting these cells, it also helps to prevent thickening of the arteries, which is also related to high blood pressure."

While this finding may be news to us, it wasn't news to prehistoric man. "This diet isn't new," says Dr. Tobian. "In fact, it's been the diet of every human being on the planet for almost 3.5 million years. The hunter-gatherer diet was high in potassium, low in sodium and fat. Evolution made humans exceedingly well adapted to that kind of diet. Strokes are really diseases of civilization." According to Dr. Tobian, people today eat only a quarter of the potassium consumed by primitive hunter-gatherers.

One way to avoid this disease of today is to go back to our roots. To do this, Dr. Tobian recommends a diet that you can hunt down and gather easily at your local supermarket. It's a diet he follows himself. "You should eat a lot of steamed vegetables," he recommends. "Don't boil them, because much of the potassium leaches into the water. And remember that by adding one baked potato, an 8-ounce glass of orange or grapefruit juice, half a melon or a glass of skim milk to what you normally eat each day, you could help lower your stroke rate by 40 percent."

STROKE
A DAY OF INTENSIVE HEALING

A.M.

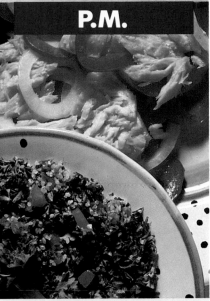

Cooked high-fiber cereal
Canned, juice-packed cut
  peaches
Vanilla low-fat yogurt

NOON

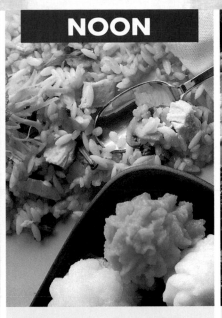

Rice pilaf with chicken bits,
  mushrooms and steamed
  spinach
Mashed carrots, turnips and
  potatoes
Chopped dried fruit
  compote
Creamy orange drink made
  with skim milk

P.M.

Chopped onions, red pep-
  pers and canned salmon
  chunks with olive oil and
  vinegar
Salad (cracked wheat, finely
  chopped tomato and
  parsley)
Banana skim-milk shake

DISASTER PLATE

Reuben sandwich (corned
  beef, cheese and sauer-
  kraut on bread dipped
  in egg batter and fried)
Dark beer

   You've just finished eating
a Reuben sandwich; now
close your eyes and listen.

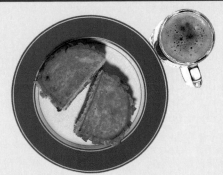

That's the sound of your
arteries slamming shut.
Corned beef is loaded with
fat and cholesterol, not to
mention the cheese, egg
batter, and the frying
process. As for beer—heavy
drinkers increase their risk
even more.

INTENSIVE HEALING RECIPES:
STROKE

Eating saturated fat can contribute to artery disease and high blood pressure. Both are risk factors for stroke. So it makes sense to limit saturated fats and to eat more fish for the special type of fat that actually combats cholesterol.

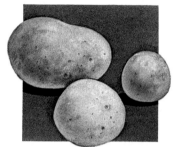

Potatoes offer potassium —a known stroke fighter.

CURRIED POTATO SALAD

1   lb. waxy potatoes
¼   cup raisins, chopped
2   scallions, minced
3   Tbsp. sliced almonds
½   tsp. curry powder, warmed
2   Tbsp. plain yogurt
1   Tbsp. chutney

Cut potatoes into 1-inch chunks, place in a large saucepan and steam until tender, about 12 minutes or more. Drain and place in a large bowl, then add raisins, scallions and almonds.

In a small bowl, combine curry powder, yogurt and chutney. Pour over potatoes and combine well. Serve warm.

Yield: 4 servings

SABLEFISH STEAK WITH BASIL AIOLI

1   lb. sablefish steak
2   Tbsp. olive oil
2   Tbsp. freshly squeezed lemon juice
¼   cup fresh basil (about 6 leaves)

Preheat the broiler or prepare the grill.

Rub fish on both sides with small amount of oil. Broil or grill until cooked through, about 5 minutes on each side for a 1-inch-thick steak.

Meanwhile, pour remaining oil into a spice grinder, mini-food processor or mortar and pestle and add lemon juice and basil. Process or grind into a smooth paste. Spoon over hot fish before serving.

Yield: 4 servings

Curried Potato Salad

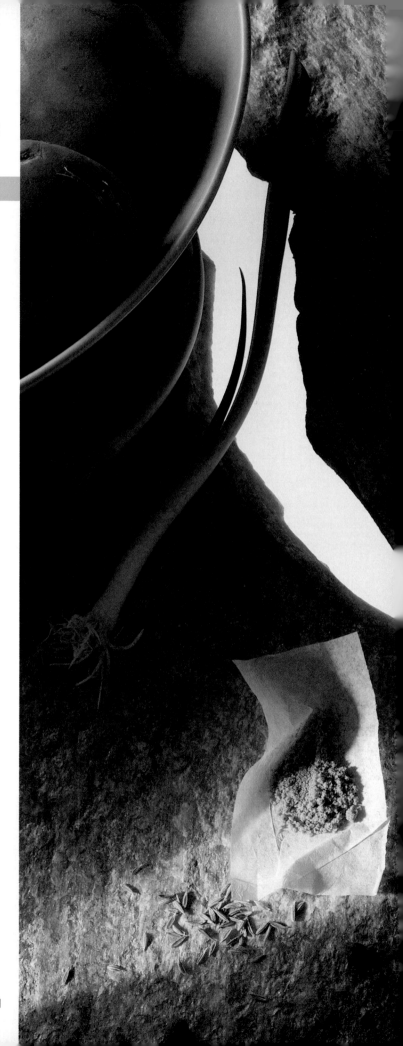

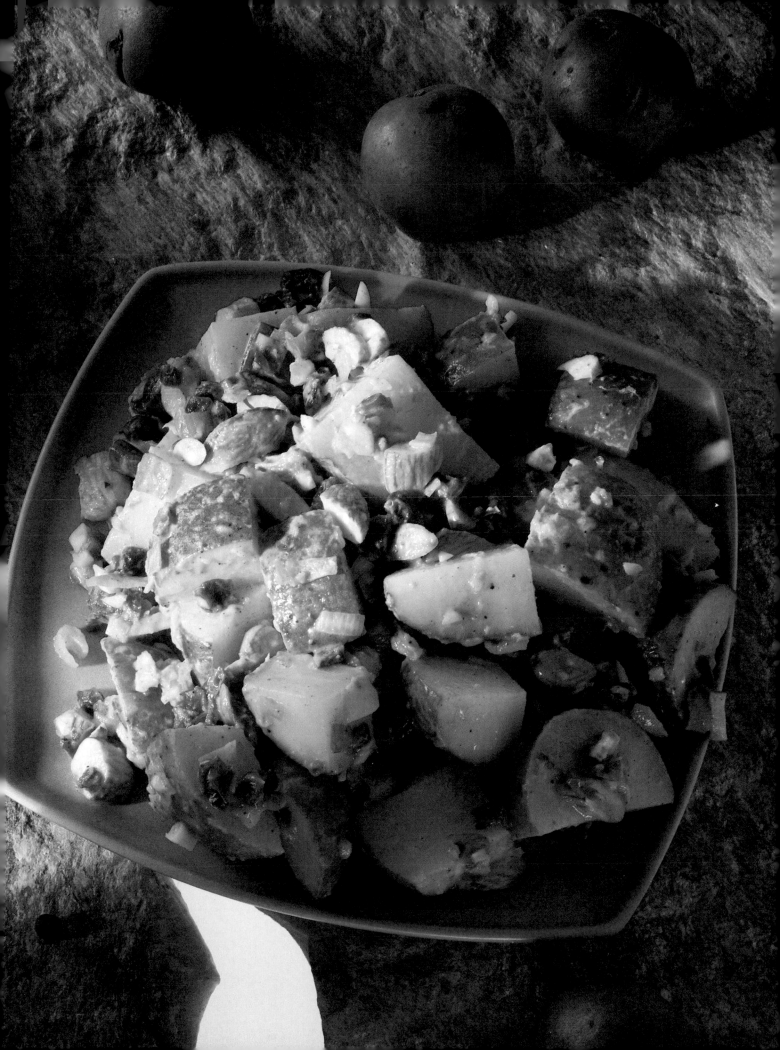

TRIGLYCERIDES

They're the Bonnie and Clyde of heart disease: cholesterol and triglycerides. We've already discussed one (see the entry on cholesterol, beginning on page 38). Let's now turn to the other.

Triglycerides do two things. They provide the body's major source of energy from fat. In fact, most of the fat and oil we eat is composed of triglyceride molecules. They are the body's main storage form of energy. Much of the fat, sugar or carbohydrates we eat that we don't quickly burn as energy is converted to triglycerides and moved through the bloodstream to be stored in chunky thighs or rounded bellies.

While traveling through the blood, triglycerides can sometimes stick to artery walls, just like cholesterol. Of the two fatty substances, however, only cholesterol has received a mountain of bad publicity, perhaps because we're less certain about the role of triglycerides in heart disease.

But this may be changing. Consider the findings of the Framingham Heart Study, a long-term health survey of a Massachusetts town. At first glance, researchers thought that, by themselves, triglycerides didn't cause heart disease. Not too long ago, however, with newer means of analysis, the same researchers came to the opposite conclusion.

"New data show that triglycerides *are* an independent risk factor for heart disease," says William Castelli, M.D., medical director of the Framingham Heart Study. "Anyone who has high blood lipids—cholesterol or triglycerides—should be considered a high-risk coronary patient."

Older women should be especially concerned about high triglyceride levels, according to these new findings. "Our recent data showed that having high triglycerides is a terrible risk factor for women." In women over age 50, says Dr. Castelli, triglycerides are "a better predictor of coronary disease than LDL [low-density lipoprotein] cholesterol."

Doctors already use triglyceride levels (measured as part of a standard cholesterol test) as a general indicator of health status. They agree that low levels are a sign of good health because they almost always occur along with low levels of other harmful fatty particles, like cholesterol. They also agree that high levels are at least indirectly associated with an increased risk of heart disease because they are invariably accompanied by high levels of other harmful blood fats.

In other words, triglycerides may do their harm independently, at least in some people. But they

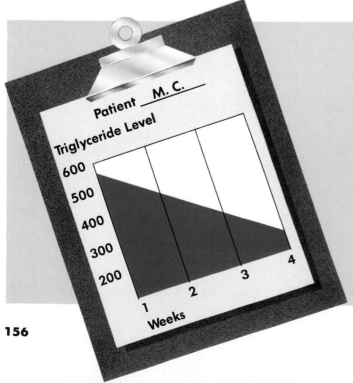

FISH OIL LOWERS TRIGLYCERIDES

There's little doubt about it: Eating fish can be good for your heart. In one British study, measured amounts of fish oil (15 grams a day or the equivalent of an 8-ounce serving of herring or mackerel) were added to the diets of five patients with high triglycerides. Four out of the five saw their levels drop dramatically in just four weeks. Patient "M. C." experienced the most dramatic drop. He went from a stratospheric 531 (milligrams of triglycerides per deciliter of blood) to a much-closer-to-earth level of 199.

almost certainly cause trouble in league with other forms of fat in the blood.

TRIM BODY, TRIM BLOOD

The more fat we have encasing our bodies, the more we have circulating in our bloodstream. That's why Don Mannerberg, M.D., author of *Aerobic Nutrition*, calls high triglycerides "a kind of internal fatness. Just as we can get fat under the layers of our skin and in our bodies, we can have fat blood, so to speak," he explains.

Triglyceride levels in the blood vary greatly from hour to hour, depending on food intake. After a large greasy or sugary meal, levels can rise dramatically and stay high for hours. Therefore, a triglycerides blood test is always done after an overnight fast. Today most doctors agree that a normal range is from 85 up to 250 (milligrams per deciliter of blood). From 250 to 500 is considered a mildly to moderately elevated level. Severely high levels, 500 and above, are usually genetic.

What should you do if you're one of the millions of Americans whose trigylcerides are moderately high, approaching 250 or more? First, have three separate blood tests to confirm the diagnosis. "I do this to make sure the lab was correct and to establish a good baseline level before beginning treatment," says Scott Grundy, M.D., Ph.D., director of the Center for Human Nutrition at the University of Texas.

His treatment, in all but the most extremely elevated cases, begins with weight loss, exercise and dietary changes, not drugs.

In many ways, fighting high triglycerides involves the same sort of measures you would follow to fight high cholesterol, like shedding excess pounds, for instance. "I can't emphasize enough how important it is to lose weight," Dr. Grundy says. "Even ten pounds can help in people who are only 20 to 30 percent overweight. Any extra energy the body has that it doesn't need turns into triglycerides. The loose calories floating around in your body that you don't burn up are made into triglycerides."

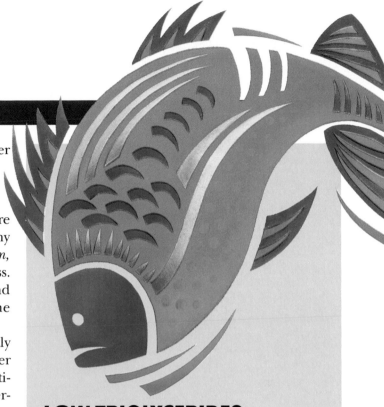

LOW TRIGLYCERIDES NATIVE TO FISH EATERS

Compared to bypass operations and artificial hearts, eating fish may seem like primitive medicine for your ticker.

But a study of African tribesmen reinforces what many studies have already shown: when you eat fish, you reel in powerful protection for your heart.

Researchers measured blood fats in two tribes that are similar in all respects except one: For the shore-dwelling Njemps, fish constitutes a substantial part of their daily diet, while the Masai generally don't eat fish. They found that the level of triglycerides was *31 percent* lower in the fish-eating tribe.

So when you go to the market, put fish at the top of your list. The catch of the day may just net you a healthier heart.

TRIGLYCERIDES RISE AFTER A MEAL

If your doctor didn't ask you to fast overnight before you took your triglycerides blood test, you'd almost certainly fail. That's because your blood fat level temporarily shoots up after most meals. Notice in the graph at the right how the average person's triglyceride level rises during the three hours following a full breakfast.

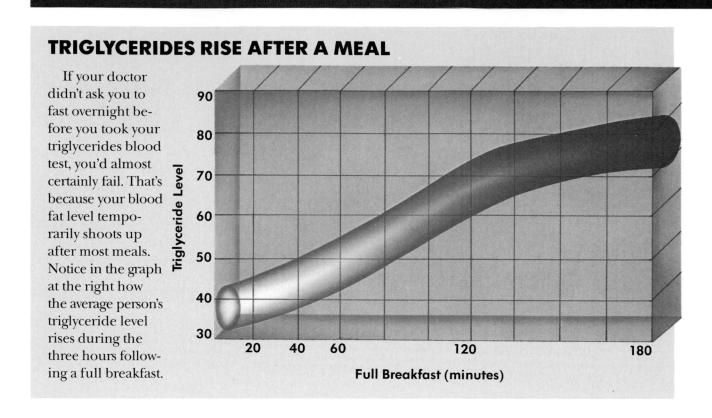

There's no doubt that the typically high-saturated-fat, high-cholesterol American diet dramatically enhances triglycerides' potential for harm. "You should make fat 35 percent or less of your calories to reduce this effect," Dr. Mannerberg says.

Sugar may be another dietary problem. Eating sugary foods will raise triglyceride levels significantly for some people, says Sheldon Reiser, Ph.D., research leader at the U.S. Department of Agriculture's Carbohydrates Nutrition Laboratory in Beltsville, Maryland.

Most likely to see this effect are people with non-insulin-dependent (Type II) diabetes or individuals with triglyceride-metabolizing problems. But other people might also want to think about keeping their sugar intake low, Dr. Reiser says. "Sugar and saturated fat work together to raise the fatty components of blood more than either would alone. It's a synergistic effect."

Some people, especially those sensitive to sugar, also have high triglyceride levels when they drink and so should also avoid alcohol, Dr. Mannerberg says.

And while you're avoiding alcohol and sugar, it may be wise to eat more fish—particularly oily fish like salmon or mackerel. "There's good evidence that fish oils lower triglyceride levels," says Dr. Mannerberg. One study found that average triglyceride levels fell from 91 to 52 in people on diets rich in fish oils.

In summary, lifestyle changes, including diet, are "the most important means of treatment of high triglycerides in most people," says Dr. Grundy. "And it's important to give these things time to work. I'd give them several months to a year." It's important to be patient and not to give up on your new lifestyle. If this doesn't work, he adds, you may turn to one of several prescription drugs currently available.

TRIGLYCERIDES
A DAY OF INTENSIVE HEALING

A.M.

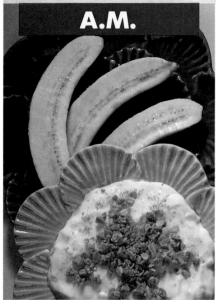

Plain low-fat yogurt with
   toasted granola and bran
Sliced banana
Orange juice

NOON

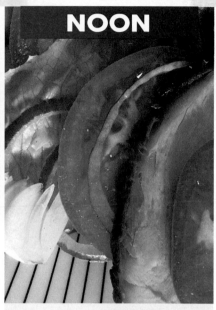

Sliced white meat turkey
Salad (romaine, tomato,
   onions and garlic) with
   olive oil dressing
Baked potato
Whole wheat pita
Watermelon wedge

P.M.

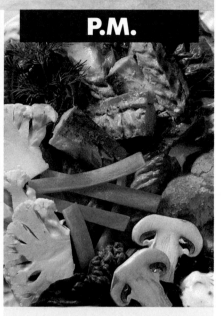

Vegetarian bean soup
Mackerel salad (canned
   mackerel, spinach,
   romaine, mushrooms,
   carrots, cauliflower and
   red onions) with low-fat
   yogurt-dill dressing
Skim milk
Fresh strawberries

DISASTER PLATE

Sour cream cheesecake
with cherry pie-filling
topping

   Triglyceride levels,
because they are so vola-
tile, are particularly fun to
play with. Here's a real fun
dish that'll send *your*

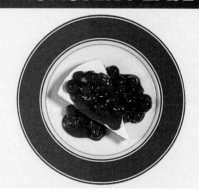

triglyceride level right into
the *Guinness Book of World
Records*. You really can't
beat it. Imagine this: All together on one tiny dessert
plate, you can get saturated
fat from the cheese, more fat
from the butter, and sugar
—lots of it. Wow!

159

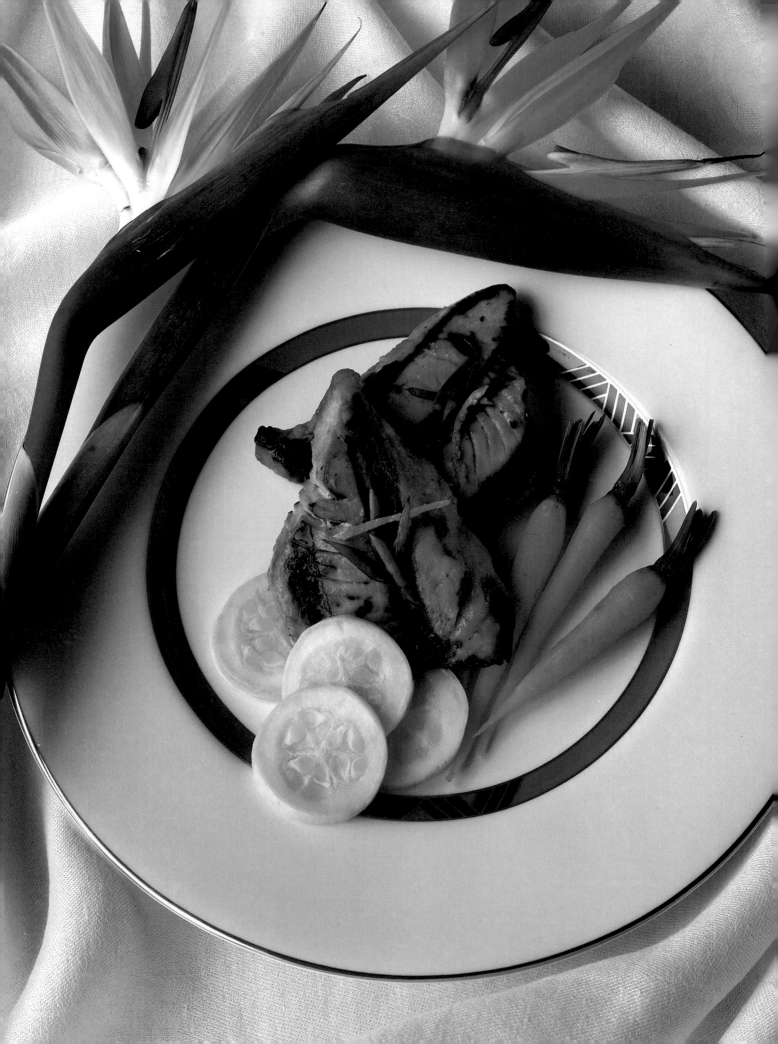

Some of the same foods that are recommended to help lower cholesterol levels may also reduce triglycerides. The following recipes offer fish, which supplies beneficial oils; rabbit, which is extremely low in fat; and garlic and onions, both of which have been shown to contribute to reduced levels of blood fats.

TUNA WITH ORANGE AND GINGER

1 Tbsp. orange marmalade
¼ cup freshly squeezed orange juice
½ tsp. finely minced peeled gingerroot
2 tsp. peanut oil
1 lb. tuna steaks
4 scallions, chopped, for garnish

In a small bowl, combine marmalade, juice, ginger and oil.

Place tuna steaks in a single layer in a Pyrex baking dish and pour juice mixture over them. Marinate for about 30 minutes.

Preheat the broiler or prepare the grill. (Grilling is a nice idea for tuna steaks because the grill marks are quite attractive.) Reserving marinade, place tuna on the broiler or grill and cook until cooked through, about 4 or 5 minutes on each side.

Meanwhile, in a small saucepan or microwave-safe dish, heat reserved marinade on the stove or in the microwave until just bubbly. Spoon over cooked tuna and sprinkle with scallions before serving. Serve with steamed baby carrots and slices of yellow squash.

Yield: 4 servings

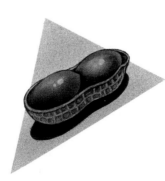

These recipes use *mono-unsaturated* peanut oil because it's healthier than saturated fat.

RABBIT SZECHUAN STYLE

1 Tbsp. peanut oil
1 rabbit (about 2 lb.), cut into 7 pieces
1½ cups chicken stock
1 Tbsp. low-sodium soy sauce
1 Tbsp. dark honey
1 tsp. finely minced gingerroot
2 cloves garlic, finely minced
1 tsp. hot pepper sauce, or to taste
2 Tbsp. tomato paste
Minced scallions, for garnish

Heat oil in a well-seasoned cast-iron skillet, or a nonstick skillet.

Add rabbit and sauté until it begins to brown, about 5 minutes.

Meanwhile, in a medium-size bowl, combine stock, soy sauce, honey, ginger, garlic, hot pepper sauce and tomato paste. Pour sauce over rabbit.

Reduce heat, cover loosely and simmer until cooked through, about 20 to 25 minutes. Sprinkle with scallions before serving. Serve with rice or thin noodles.

Yield: 4 servings

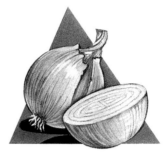

Pungent with flavor and packed with power, the onion may be good medicine for reducing blood fats like triglycerides.

CARROT AND SWEET ONION RELISH

2 sweet onions, chopped
2 carrots, chopped
1 tsp. fresh rosemary, chopped
1 bay leaf
⅓ cup cider vinegar
⅓ cup water

Combine all ingredients in a medium-size bowl, stir well and cover. Refrigerate overnight.

Before serving, remove bay leaf and drain liquid. Serve as an accompaniment to grilled poultry.

Yield: 4 servings

Tuna with Orange and Ginger

ULCERS

It could be worse. You could be living in 1918 when the recommended treatment for a peptic ulcer was feeding the patient via the rectum. Make you lose your appetite?

Today physicians are recommending much more palatable treatments. "I usually tell my patients to eat whatever they want except for things that have given them an upset stomach in the past," says Alan Adelman, M.D., assistant professor at the University of Maryland School of Medicine and a researcher of abdominal pain. No tasteless diet? No ban on spicy food?

"The bland diet that was used years ago was never really documented to be effective and has gone by the wayside," says Dr. Adelman, who adds, "Spicy foods are not held to be the culprit anymore."

Under the right conditions, even peppery foods may be okay if they don't cause discomfort. "It's been shown that an irritant, introduced in low doses over a period of time, actually helps the stomach build up a defense against other substances that would tend to damage it," says David Earnest, M.D., professor of medicine at the University of Arizona Science

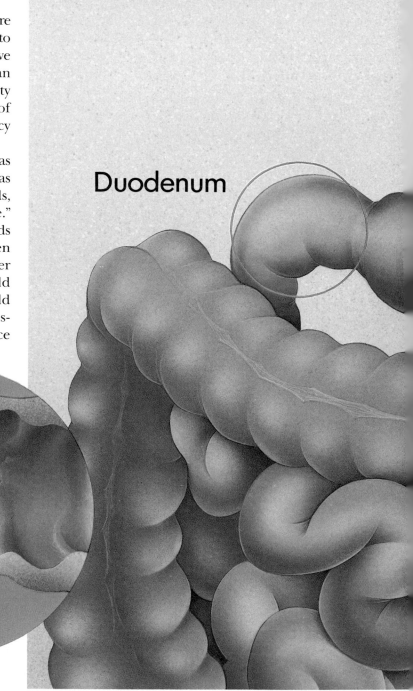

Duodenum

A duodenal ulcer may result from excess acid that flows from the stomach into the duodenum. Another factor contributing to ulcers can be damage to the protective mucous lining of the stomach or duodenum. These factors may be related in that the excess acid may be the cause of damage to the mucous lining.

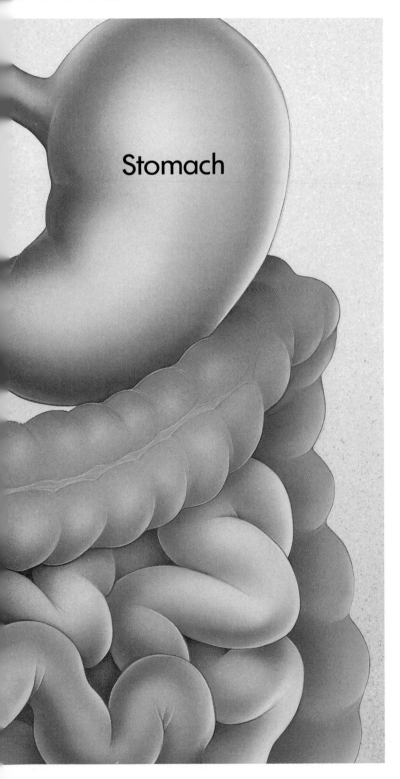

Stomach

Center and chairman of the Committee on Patient Care for the American Gastroenterological Association. He says research has proven that treating ulcers with diets just doesn't work. "Diet was written off ten years ago as a primary mode of ulcer treatment. People treated with diets alone took twice as long to heal as people today, who are treated with modern, effective medication."

UDDER NONSENSE

Many people suffering with a peptic ulcer (that is, an ulcer located in the stomach and duodenum) drink milk to ease the pain. But drinking milk may be ill-advised, says Richard McCallum, M.D., professor of medicine and chief of gastroenterology at the University of Virginia School of Medicine. "Drinking lots of milk is out. Initially it may neutralize some acid and you may feel better, but the calcium and protein in it actually stimulate acid to be released. You get a 'rebound effect'—30 or more minutes after drinking milk, your acid level actually goes up. We counsel patients to not rely on drinking milk to relieve their pain, but to drink antacids or eat crackers or some other food known to buffer acid. No acid, no ulcer."

DISCOVERING THE CAUSE—AND CURE

Most everyone agrees that stomach acid causes ulcers. But one renegade from Australia—gastroenterologist Barry Marshall, M.D.—thinks he's found another cause: bacteria.

In this new and developing research, Dr. Marshall tested hundreds of patients with duodenal ulcers and found in most of them a type of bacteria that he calls *Campylobacter pyloridis*. When he treated those patients with bismuth (an ingredient in Pepto-Bismol), he found that not only did the bacteria disappear but so did the ulcers. When he combined bismuth with an antibacterial drug, 75 percent of the ulcers cleared up. He even went so far as swallowing a colony of the bacteria, developing gastritis and then curing it with a dose of bismuth and antibiotic. That time, it really was something he ate.

VEGETARIANISM

He's a massive man, with sheets of muscle covering his chest and ropes of sinew wrapped around his arms and legs.

Like most bodybuilders, he's deeply tanned. Bronzed skin brings out the separation between muscles that these sculptors of the human form call *definition.*

When he works his muscles, that definition starts to show. The heart pumps blood into every straining muscle until the most minute striations in biceps and pectorals can be seen through the skin.

Bill Pearl, in the jargon of the gym, is *ripped.*

But that isn't what makes him unique. This 57-year-old man has 19-inch arms and a chest so thick that bench-pressing 400 pounds is no sweat at all. He's been known to stand up with 550 pounds of steel on his back, and six days a week he growls his way through morning workouts that last for three hours.

What makes this red-blooded epitome of the ideal bodybuilder so unique is not what he does but what he eats. Bill Pearl looks like a carnivore but eats like the gentlest of God's creatures: He's been a vegetarian for more than 20 years.

THE BLIND LEADING THE BLIND

"It's an absolute myth that weight lifters or other athletes have to eat meat to stay healthy and get big," Pearl says today.

"I did it when I started out only because that's what all the top people in bodybuilding were doing —and even though it conflicted with everything the real experts in nutrition were telling me. It was a case of the blind leading the blind."

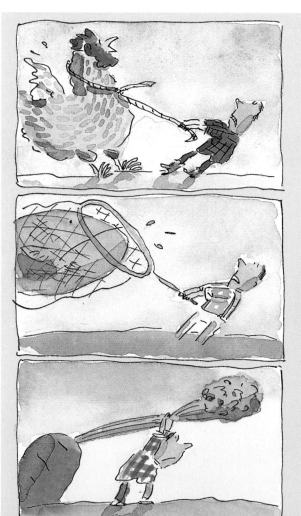

THE GRADUAL VEGETARIAN

Making the change to vegetarianism can be a painless, pleasant experience if you follow the advice of Lisa Tracy, author of *The Gradual Vegetarian.*

First, analyze your diet to find out what you're eating and why you're eating it. The goal: to identify eating and other habits that don't fit in with your goal, and those that do.

Next, map a strategy. This is where you decide what changes to make and when you're going to make them—replacing red meat with chicken, for example. You also locate the resources (like good grocery stores) you'll need to make the changes.

Finally, start doing it. But remember Tracy's first principle: Do it in stages. First, eliminate red meat only. Second, drop poultry from your diet. Third, drop the fish—and pat yourself on the back for officially achieving vegetarianism. And finally, don't worry about time. Tracy says that like giving up smoking, making the transition to vegetarianism may take several tries over several years. Just stick with it.

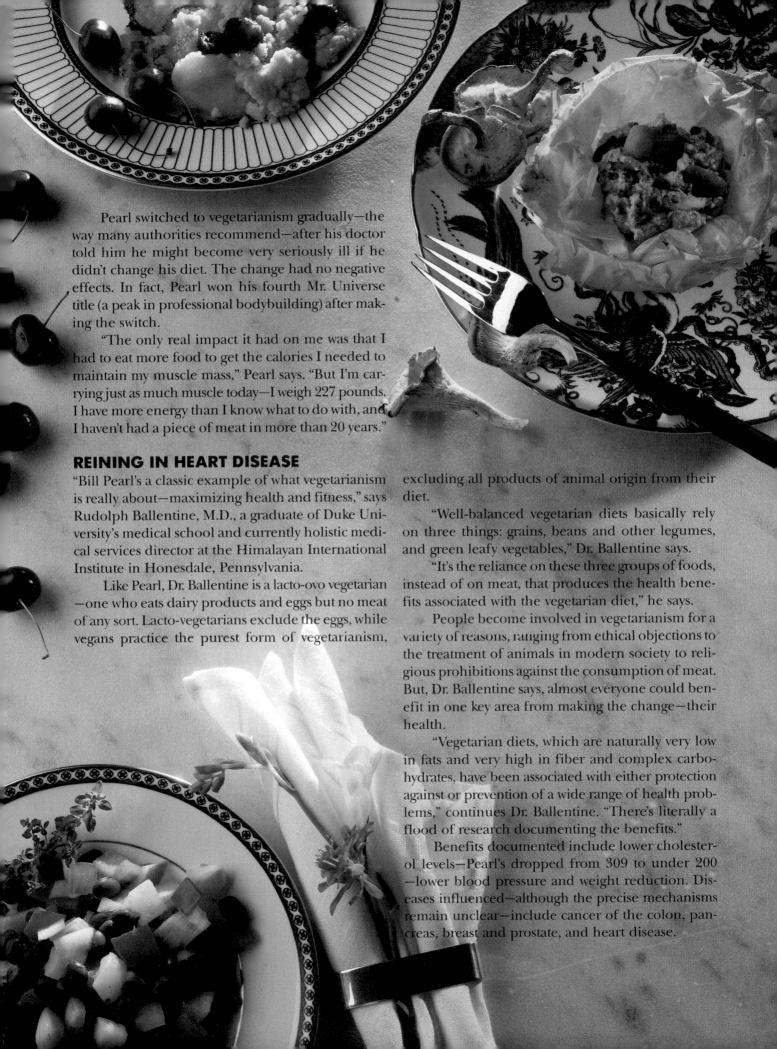

Pearl switched to vegetarianism gradually—the way many authorities recommend—after his doctor told him he might become very seriously ill if he didn't change his diet. The change had no negative effects. In fact, Pearl won his fourth Mr. Universe title (a peak in professional bodybuilding) after making the switch.

"The only real impact it had on me was that I had to eat more food to get the calories I needed to maintain my muscle mass," Pearl says. "But I'm carrying just as much muscle today—I weigh 227 pounds. I have more energy than I know what to do with, and I haven't had a piece of meat in more than 20 years."

REINING IN HEART DISEASE

"Bill Pearl's a classic example of what vegetarianism is really about—maximizing health and fitness," says Rudolph Ballentine, M.D., a graduate of Duke University's medical school and currently holistic medical services director at the Himalayan International Institute in Honesdale, Pennsylvania.

Like Pearl, Dr. Ballentine is a lacto-ovo vegetarian —one who eats dairy products and eggs but no meat of any sort. Lacto-vegetarians exclude the eggs, while vegans practice the purest form of vegetarianism, excluding all products of animal origin from their diet.

"Well-balanced vegetarian diets basically rely on three things: grains, beans and other legumes, and green leafy vegetables," Dr. Ballentine says.

"It's the reliance on these three groups of foods, instead of on meat, that produces the health benefits associated with the vegetarian diet," he says.

People become involved in vegetarianism for a variety of reasons, ranging from ethical objections to the treatment of animals in modern society to religious prohibitions against the consumption of meat. But, Dr. Ballentine says, almost everyone could benefit in one key area from making the change—their health.

"Vegetarian diets, which are naturally very low in fats and very high in fiber and complex carbohydrates, have been associated with either protection against or prevention of a wide range of health problems," continues Dr. Ballentine. "There's literally a flood of research documenting the benefits."

Benefits documented include lower cholesterol levels—Pearl's dropped from 309 to under 200 —lower blood pressure and weight reduction. Diseases influenced—although the precise mechanisms remain unclear—include cancer of the colon, pancreas, breast and prostate, and heart disease.

"A diet that includes meat has been associated in some studies with heart attacks. Meat eaters in these studies suffered 3½ times the number of heart attacks that their vegetarian counterparts—men between the ages of 44 and 65—did," Dr. Ballentine says. "The implications for this country, where up to 40 percent of the population still dies from heart disease, are tremendous."

SENSIBLE SUBSTITUTES

Going meatless can mean giving up your primary source of certain nutrients like iron. But a little knowledge will help you replace them with nutritious nonmeat sources. The list below tells you what's where.

NUTRIENT	SOURCES
CALCIUM	Dairy products, dark leafy greens, legumes, most nuts and seeds, molasses, figs, apricots and dates
IRON	Legumes (especially soybeans) and soy products other than soy oil, dark leafy greens, dried fruits, whole and enriched grains, and molasses
PROTEIN	Legumes, grains, nuts, seeds, eggs and dairy products
RIBOFLAVIN	Dairy products, eggs, whole and enriched grains, brewer's yeast, dark leafy greens and legumes
VITAMIN B$_{12}$	Dairy products, eggs, yeast, foods fortified with B$_{12}$, and supplements
VITAMIN D	Fortified milk, fortified soy milk, exposure of skin to sunshine
ZINC	Eggs, cheese, legumes, nuts, wheat germ, whole grains and some kinds of brewer's yeast

A DIET THAT'S EASY TO FOLLOW

Bill Pearl, and others like him, pretty thoroughly debunk the popular image of vegetarians—distinctly scrawny, probably pale, definitely weird. But many people reject vegetarianism for another reason—complexity. One of the strongest myths circulating about meatless eating is that you place your health at risk unless you mix and match foods just right.

"I think that's absolute nonsense," says Frank Sacks, M.D., a researcher at Harvard Medical School's Channing Laboratory. "As long as you eat reasonable quantities from all the major food groups allowed, the average adult has nothing to worry about."

Not that vegetarianism is risk-free—it isn't. Dr. Ballentine says that certain nutrients—iron, for example, and calcium—may pose problems. Iron from plant sources and bran, commonly given to older people for constipation, can hijack calcium and carry it out of the body. The result? Painful leg cramps from a lack of calcium.

But Ballentine says there are solutions that reduce the risk—and they're *not* always supplements.

"A multivitamin and mineral supplement isn't a bad idea, but it's no substitute for paying attention to what you eat and how you prepare it. One example: You can increase your iron four times or so just by cooking in iron pots. Eat a vitamin C-rich food such as tomatoes with an iron-rich food, and you may increase your iron absorption by four times."

But knowledge in one particular area probably benefits the vegetarian more than any other. Dr. Ballentine says that proper *cooking* skills minimize problems with going meat-free. "It's really important," he says.

"Proper seasoning can make meatless foods much more attractive to the American palate and improve the nutritional content. Good cooking techniques like microwaving help retain the food's nutritional value. And little things like peeling to reduce your total fiber can essentially eliminate problems like gas. Whatever you do, *don't* add bran. You'll get plenty of fiber without it."

VEGETARIANISM GONE WRONG

It ain't working: The wonderful things your vegetarian friends said you would experience—weight loss, more energy, less fatigue—just aren't happening. And you want to know why.

Chances are the answer's simple: You've eliminated meat but everything else about your diet has remained the same. It's still loaded with fat, sugar and unhealthy amounts of salt. In other words, you aren't really a vegetarian.

"There's more to it than just giving up meat," says Rudolph Ballentine, M.D. "It's easy, in fact, to technically fit the definition of a vegetarian and still eat so badly you're at risk of malnutrition."

How? By eating the wrong foods or foods prepared the wrong way. An example of wrong food might be a grilled cheese sandwich on white bread. It's a meatless lunch, but it's loaded with fat and salt. Examples of foods prepared the wrong way include vegetables that are breaded and fried, or a baked potato served under a mound of sour cream.

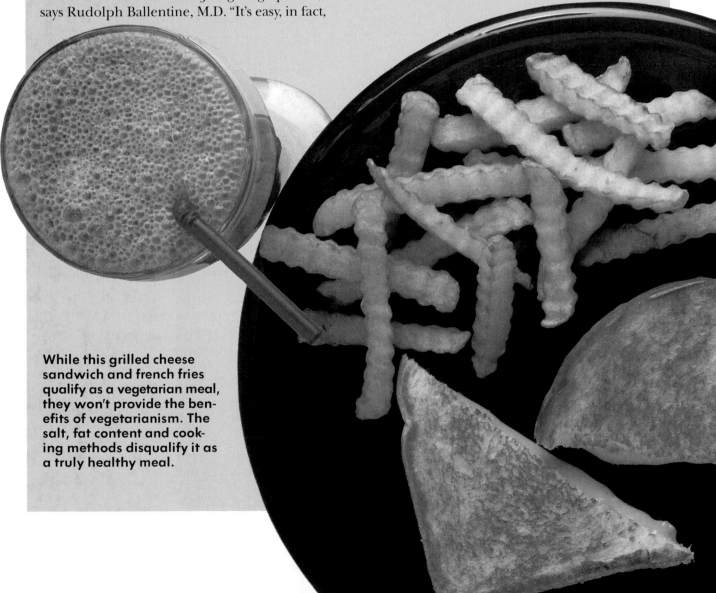

While this grilled cheese sandwich and french fries qualify as a vegetarian meal, they won't provide the benefits of vegetarianism. The salt, fat content and cooking methods disqualify it as a truly healthy meal.

INTENSIVE HEALING RECIPES:
VEGETARIANISM

Some people may think of vegetarian meals as salad and more salad. Here are two recipes that provide stick-to-your-ribs dishes. Fusilli with Fresh Tomato Sauce and Peppers with Cracked Wheat and Saffron are colorful, zesty main dishes that pack plenty of nutrition. And think of the health benefits!

FUSILLI WITH FRESH TOMATO SAUCE

5	fresh tomatoes, peeled, seeded and juiced, or 10 canned plum tomatoes, seeded and juiced
8	pitted green olives
¼	cup fresh basil (about 6 leaves)
	Juice and pulp of 1 lemon
1	shallot
1	Tbsp. olive oil
1½	cups uncooked fusilli
	Freshly grated Parmesan cheese
	Basil sprigs, for garnish

Place tomatoes, olives, basil, lemon, shallot and oil in a food processor or blender and process until well combined but not quite smooth. Cover and set aside for about 2 hours to let flavors blend.

Cook fusilli until tender. Drain well, place in a large bowl and toss with Parmesan and tomato sauce. Garnish with basil and serve at room temperature.

Yield: 4 servings

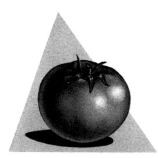

Although low in calories, a tomato offers lots of vitamins A and C, as well as potassium.

PEPPERS WITH CRACKED WHEAT AND SAFFRON

½	cup medium-coarse cracked wheat
4	bell peppers, cored and seeded
1	Tbsp. olive oil
¼	cup chopped onions
½	tsp. saffron threads
½	tsp. dried thyme
2	cloves garlic, finely minced
¼	cup part-skim ricotta
1	egg

Measure wheat into a medium-size bowl and add boiling water to cover. Set aside until wheat has absorbed the water, about 20 to 30 minutes. If wheat does not soften, add a bit more water.

Blanch peppers in boiling water until just tender, about 4 minutes. Set aside to cool.

Heat oil in a large sauté pan. Then add onions, saffron, thyme and garlic and sauté until onions are tender, about 5 minutes. Do not allow garlic to burn.

Preheat the oven to 350°F.

Place ricotta and egg in a food processor or blender and process until smooth. Add onion mixture and wheat to ricotta mixture and combine well. Divide filling among peppers.

Place filled peppers in a baking dish and bake until filling is firm and cooked through, about 20 to 25 minutes. Serve hot.

Yield: 4 servings

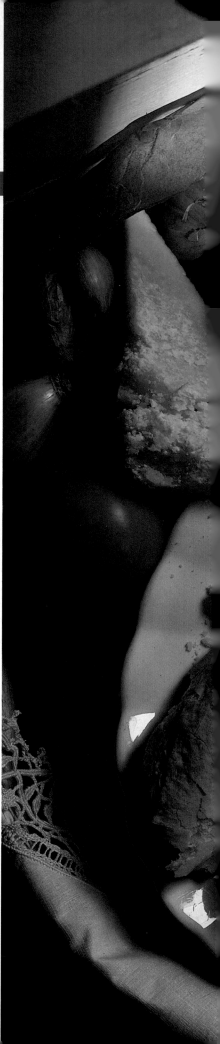

Fusilli with Fresh Tomato Sauce

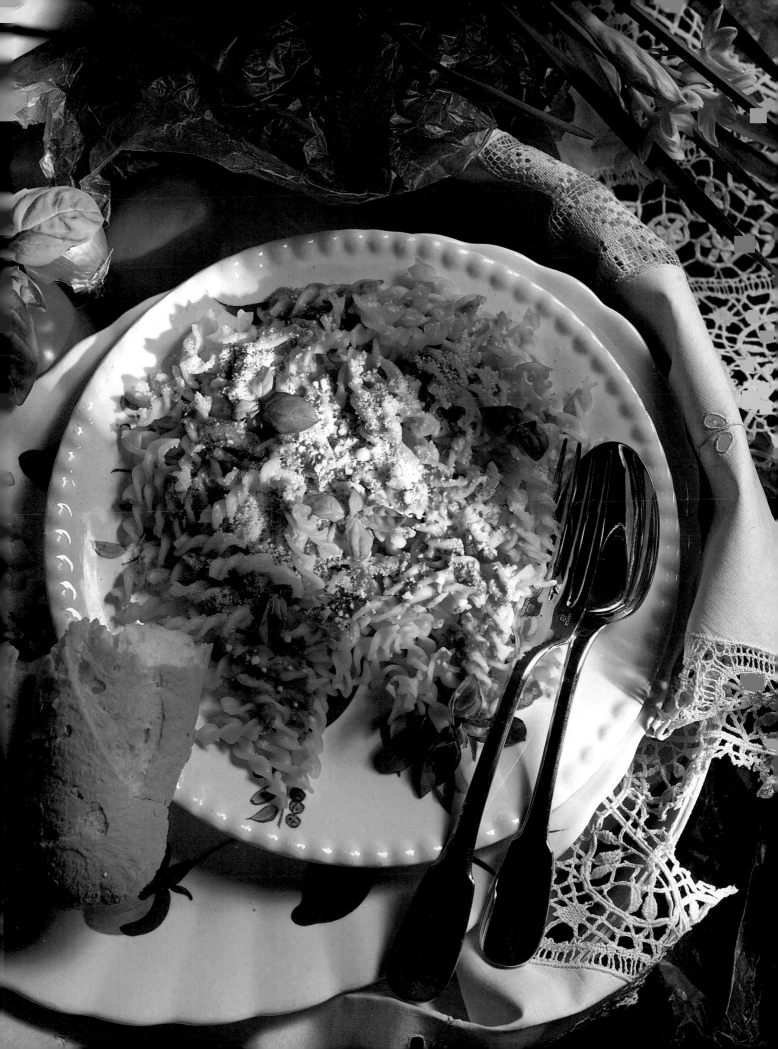

SOURCES & CREDITS

SOURCE NOTES

Allergies

page 10

"Food Allergies Change with Age" adapted from the Food Study Program of the National Asthma Center and committee member Hugh Sampson, M.D.

page 13

"Welcome to the Allergy Family" adapted from *Clinical Ecology*, by Lawrence Dickey (Springfield, Ill.: Charles C. Thomas, 1976) and *An Alternative Approach to Allergies*, by Theron Randolph and Ralph Moss (New York: Harper & Row, 1980).

Anemia

page 20

"Best Food Sources of Iron" adapted from Agriculture Handbook Nos. 8-5, 8-9, 8-11, 8-12, 8-13, 8-15, 8-16, 456 (Washington, D.C.: U.S. Department of Agriculture).

Arthritis

page 22

"An Ocean of Relief" adapted from "Fish-Oil Fatty Acid Supplementation in Active Rheumatoid Arthritis," *Annals of Internal Medicine,* April 1987.

Cholesterol

page 41

"Relative Risk" adapted from "Nutritional Contributors to Cardiovascular Disease in the Elderly," by W. B. Kannel, M.D., F.A.C.E., Framingham Heart Study, *American Journal of Cardiology,* 52:12B, 1983.

page 44

"Where's the Pectin?" compiled from information provided by Nutrient Data Research Branch, U.S. Department of Agriculture, and *Metabolic Effects of Dietary Pectins Related to Human Health,* by Sheldon Reiser (Beltsville, Md.: Carbohydrate Nutrition Laboratory, Beltsville Human Nutrition Research Center, Agricultural Research Service, U.S. Department of Agriculture, 1986) and *Effects of Pectin on Human Metabolism,* by Sheldon Reiser and Kay Behall (Beltsville, Md.: Carbohydrate Nutrition Laboratory, Beltsville Human Nutrition Research Center, Agricultural Research Service, U.S. Department of Agriculture, 1986) and *Introductory Foods,* 5th ed., by Osee Hughes and Marion Bennion (London: Macmillan Company, Collier-Macmillan Ltd., 1970).

Diverticulosis

page 64

"How Things Change" compiled by Marvin Schuster, M.D., Chief of Digestive Medicine, Francis Scott Key Medical Center, Baltimore, Maryland.

Fringe Diets and Beyond

page 72

"The Standard Macrobiotic Diet" reprinted from *Macrobiotic Diet: Balancing Your Eating in Harmony with the Changing Environment and Personal Needs,* by Michio and Aveline Kushi, edited by Alex Jack (Tokyo and New York: Japan Publications, Inc., 1985, p. 50).

Gout

page 77

"Purine Sources" adapted from *Food, Nutrition and Diet Therapy,* by M. Krause, B.S., M.S., R.D., and K. Mahan M.S., R.D. (Philadelphia: W. B. Saunders Co., 1984) and *Food Values of Portions Commonly Used,* 14th Ed., by Jean Pennington, Ph.D., R.D., and Helen Nichols Church, B.S. (Philadelphia: J. B. Lippincott Co., 1985).

Heart Disease

page 82

"Rating the Fats" adapted from *The New American Diet,* by Sonja L. Connor, M.S., R.D., and William E. Connor, M.D. (New York: Simon and Schuster, 1986, pp. 74–75).

High Blood Pressure

page 91

Alcohol consumption and blood pressure chart adapted from "Alcohol Consumption and Blood Pressure: Kaiser-Permanente Multiphasic Health Examination Data," by Arthur L. Klatsky, M.D., Gary D. Friedman, M.D., M.S., Abraham B. Siegelaub, M.S., and Marie J. Gerard, M.D., of Department of Medicine, Kaiser-Permanente Medical Center and Department of Medical Methods Research, Kaiser-Permanente Medical Care Program. *The New England Journal of Medicine,* May 26, 1977, p. 1196.

Natural Food Advocates

page 127

"A Sprouting Sampler" adapted from "Super Nutrition from Sprouts," *The Hippocrates Diet and Health Program,* by Ann Wigmore (Wayne, N.J.: Avery Publishing Group, Inc., 1983, pp. 80–83).

Osteoporosis

page 134

"The Best Food Sources of Calcium" adapted from Agriculture Handbook Nos. 8-1, 8-11, 8-12, 8-15, 8-16, 456 (Washington, D.C.: U.S. Department of Agriculture).

Recuperation

page 147

"Hospital Food Flunks" reprinted from "Hospital Malnutrition: A 33-Hospital Screening Study," by Savitri K. Kamath, Ph.D., R.D., Marilyn Lawler, Ph.D., R.D., Alice E. Smith, M.S., R.D., Theresa Kalat, R.D. and Ronald Olson, Ph.D., *Journal of the American Dietetic Association,* February 1986, v. 86, No. 2, pp. 203–06.

Stroke

page 151

"Best Potassium Picks" adapted from Agriculture Handbook Nos. 8, 8-1, 8-9, 8-10, 8-11, 8-12, 8-13, 8-15, 8-16, 456 (Washington, D.C.: U.S. Department of Agriculture)
and
The Calcium Bible, by Patricia Hausman (New York: Rawson Associates, 1985)
and
Information supplied by Nutrient Data Research Branch, U.S. Department of Agriculture, Washington, D.C.

Triglycerides

page 156

"Fish Oil Lowers Triglycerides" adapted from "Triglyceride-Lowering Effect of Marine Polyunsaturates in Patients with Hypertriglyceridemia," by Thomas A. B. Sanders, David R. Sullivan, Jonathan Reeve and Gilbert R. Thompson, *Arteriosclerosis,* September/October 1985.

page 158

"Triglycerides Rise after a Meal" adapted from "Total Cholesterol, High Density Lipoprotein-Cholesterol and Triglycerides after a Standardized High-Fat Meal," by D. S. Thelle, D. G. Cramp, Ila Patel, Mary Walker, Jean W. Marr and A. G. Shaper, *Human Nutrition: Clinical Nutrition,* September 1982, v. 36c, No. 6, p. 469.

PHOTOGRAPHY CREDITS

Cover: Alison Miksch

Staff Photographers: Candace Billman: pp. 11; 25; 126, left. Angelo M. Caggiano: pp. 9; 30–31, top; 69; 107; 138–39; 151. Carl Doney: pp. 76–77; 109; 136; 150; 160; 168–69. Joe Griffin: pp. 7; 128–29. Donna M. Hornberger: pp. 15; 21, bottom; 33; 42; 45, bottom; 50; 53; 70; 81; 82–83; 100; 102; 103; 105; 153; 167. Mitchell T. Mandel: pp. 112; 132–33. Alison Miksch: pp. 2; 28–29; 37; 49; 72; 89; 94; 116, bottom left; 165. Margaret Skrovanek: p. 75. Christie C. Tito: pp. 16–17; 21, top; 23; 40; 45, top; 86–87; 93; 101; 110; 114–117 (except 116, bottom left); 123; 135; 159. Sally Shenk Ullman: pp. 6, left; 34–35; 46–47; 97; 154–55.

Other Photographers: Art Resource: p. 74. Julian Baum: pp. 142–43 (except 142, top left). Focus on Sports: p. 90. Lee Foster: p. 55. Marilynne Herbert: p. 131. Meg Landsman: p. 73. Lou Manna: p. 6, right; 145. Lyn Schneider Studio/The Stock Market: p. 43. Patricia Lynn Seip: p. 30, bottom left. Tom Tracy: p. 99. Bruce Vandale: p. 141.

Additional Photographs Courtesy of: Dr. James Anderson: p. 19. Denis Burkitt: p. 27. Feingold Assoc. of the U.S.: p. 71. Health Service/Santa Barbara, Calif.: p. 121. Viktoras Kulvinskas: p. 126, right. Norwalk Press: p. 125, top. Norwalk Sales and Service: p. 125, bottom. Pritikin Longevity Center: p. 142, top left.

Photographic Stylists: Heidi Actor: pp. 46–47; 168–69. Barbara Fritz: pp. 35; 112; 154–55. Kathryn Hanuschak: p. 72. Mary Hart: pp. 86–87; 160. Renee R. Keith: pp. 138–39; 151. Marianne G. Laubach: pp. 16–17; 21, top; 23; 28–29; 33; 40; 93; 100–101; 102; 105; 135; 136. Kay Seng Lichthardt: pp. 37; 45, top; 48; 72; 89; 94; 109; 165. Debra Lush: p. 107. Pamela Simpson: pp. 97; 110; 132–33. Kathryn E. Sommons: pp. 15; 21, bottom; 33; 45, top; 53; 105; 128–29; 135; 153; 159; 167.

ILLUSTRATION CREDITS

Laura Cornell: pp. 6; 13; 66; 67; 133; 164. Mellisa Edmonds: pp. 18; 22; 41; 59; 98; 144; 156; 158. Kathi Ember: pp. 10; 16; 34; 37; 47; 48; 77; 88; 92; 95; 106; 109; 111; 113; 119; 137; 138–39; 147; 154; 157; 161; 168. Leslie Flis: pp. 85; 91. Narda Lebo: pp. 7; 38; 62–63; 65; 104; 162–63. Stephen Moscowitz: pp. 24; 51; 78–79; 134. Susan Rosenberger: pp. 36; 57; 60–61; 149.

INDEX

Note: Page references in **boldface** indicate tables. References in *italic* indicate illustrations.

Dieting tips, 138–39, 144–45
Diverticulitis, 50, 51, *65*
Diverticulosis, 51–52, 64–65
Doctors, 118–19

E

Eggs, 40, **83,** 84
Ehret, Arnold, 122
Energy, 66–67
Enteritis, regional, 146
Epilepsy, macrobiotics and, 73
Erection problems, 101
Esophageal cancer, cured foods
   and, 30
Estrogen, calcium and, 133
Exercise
   allergies induced by, 12
   cholesterol and, 41
   constipation and, 52
   diabetes and, 59
   dieting and, 145
   malnutrition and, 147
   Pritikin diet and, 141
Eyesight, poor, rice diet and, 108

F

Fasting, 75
Fat(s)
   cancer and, 29, 30
   cholesterol and, 41
   diabetes and, 59, 60
   fibrocystic breast disease
     and, 68
   heart disease and, 80, 83, 84
   high blood pressure and, 91
   impotence and, 101
   indigestion from, 103
   Pritikin diet and, 140, 141
   Rating the Fats, **82–83**
   saturated, 39, 40, 41, 42, 80,
     82–83
   stroke and, 152
   triglycerides and, 157, 158
   types of, 41
Fatigue, 66. *See also* Anemia
Fatty acids. *See* Omega-3 fatty acids
Feingold diet, 71
Fiber, 18, 26–27
   cancer and, 29–30, 30–31
   cholesterol and, 42, 43–44, 84

constipation and, 52
diabetes and, 19, 26, 59, 60
diverticulosis and, 64–65
fibrocystic disease and, 68
intestinal gas from, 104
Fibrocystic breast disease, 68–69
Fish, 40–41, 42, 82, **83,** 157
Fish oil(s)
   arthritis treated by, 22–23
   cancer and, 32
   cholesterol lowered by, 42,
     84–85
   high blood pressure and, 91
   triglycerides lowered by, 156
Fistulas, 146
Folate, 20, 98–99
Food(s)
   craving for, 14
   healing, 114–17
   hospital, 147
   natural, advocates of, 120–27
   sprouted, **127**
   versus supplements, nutrition
     from, 85
Food allergies, 10, 11–12, 23–24
Food colorings, 71
Food combinations, 124
Food groups, 128–29
Food labels, 84
Food preparation. *See* Cooking
  methods
Fruit(s)
   cancer and, 31–32
   cystitis and, 54
   diabetes and, 61
   headaches and, 79
   heart disease and, 84
   stroke and, 152

G

Gangrene, as complication of
  diabetes, 59
Garlic, 42, 81
Gas, stomach and intestinal, 103–4
Gastritis, 163
Gingivitis, 57
Gluten, 36
Gout, 76–77
   Purine Sources, **77**

Grains
   allergies to, 11, 12
   celiac disease and, 36
   diverticulosis and, 65
Guar gum, cholesterol reduced
  by, 84
Gum disease, 57

H

HDL cholesterol, 39, 41, 43, 81,
  84, 85
Headaches, 71, 78–79
Healing, psychology of, 144–45
Heart attack, 38, 42, 44, 80, 166
Heartburn. *See* Indigestion
Heart disease, 26, 80–89
   as complication of diabetes, 59
   diets to treat, 74, 108, 140, 141
   healing foods for, 81, 116
   from high blood pressure, 90
   intensive healing recipes for, 88
   Rating the Fats, **82–83**
   triglycerides and, 156
   vegetarianism and, 165
Herbs, sleep induced by, 107
High blood pressure, 90–95, 144, 145
   blindness from, 90
   A Day of Intensive Healing
     for, 93
   diets to treat, 74, 90–91, 108,
     140, 142, 165
   Disaster Plate for, 93
   healing foods for, 116
   impotence and, 101
   intensive healing recipes for, 95
   nightshades and, 70
   obesity and, 76, 77
   potassium and, 119
   sodium contributing to, 152
   stroke and, 151
   from yohimbine, 100
High-density lipoproteins. *See* HDL
  cholesterol
Hives, 12, 14
Hormones, effect on breasts, 68
Hospitals, malnutrition in, 146, 147
Hyperactivity, in children, 71
Hypertension. *See* High blood
  pressure
Hypoglycemia, headaches from, 78

Rodale Press, Inc., publishes PREVENTION®, the better health magazine.
For information on how to order your subscription,
write to PREVENTION®, Emmaus, PA 18098.